T0259059

Update in Preventive Cardiology

Editor

DOUGLAS S. JACOBY

MEDICAL CLINICS
OF NORTH AMERICA

www.medical.theclinics.com

Consulting Editor
JACK ENDE

March 2022 • Volume 106 • Number 2

ELSEVIER

1600 John F. Kennedy Boulevard • Suite 1800 • Philadelphia, Pennsylvania, 19103-2899

http://www.theclinics.com

MEDICAL CLINICS OF NORTH AMERICA Volume 106, Number 2
March 2022 ISSN 0025-7125, ISBN-13: 978-0-323-84912-8

Editor: Katerina Heidhausen
Developmental Editor: Arlene Campos

Medical Clinics of North America (ISSN 0025-7125) is published bimonthly by Elsevier Inc., 360 Park Avenue South, New York, NY 10010-1710. Months of publication are January, March, May, July, September, and November. Business and editorial offices: 1600 John F. Kennedy Boulevard, Suite 1800, Philadelphia, PA 19103-2899. Periodicals postage paid at New York, NY, and additional mailing offices. Subscription prices are USD $316.00 per year (US individuals), $956.00 per year (US institutions), $100.00 per year (US Students), $396.00 per year (Canadian individuals), $1,004.00 per year (Canadian institutions), $200.00 per year for (foreign students), $100.00 per year for (Canadian students), $439.00 per year (foreign individuals), and $1,004.00 per year (foreign institutions). To receive student/resident rate, orders must be accompanied by name of affiliated institution, date of term, and the signature of program/residency coordinator on institution letterhead. Orders will be billed at individual rate until proof of status is received. Foreign air speed delivery is included in all Clinics' subscription prices. All prices are subject to change without notice. **POSTMASTER:** Send address changes to *Medical Clinics of North America*, Elsevier Health Sciences Division, Subscription Customer Service, 3251 Riverport Lane, Maryland Heights, MO 63043. **Customer Service: Telephone: 1-800-654-2452** (U.S. and Canada); **1-314-447-8871** (outside U.S. and Canada). **Fax: 314-447-8029. E-mail: journalscustomerserviceusa@ elsevier.com** (for print support); **journalsonlinesupport-usa@elsevier.com** (for online support).

Reprints. For copies of 100 or more of articles in this publication, please contact the Commercial Reprints Department, Elsevier Inc., 360 Park Avenue South, New York, NY 10010-1710. Tel.: 212-633-3874; Fax: 212-633-3820; E-mail: reprints@elsevier.com.

Medical Clinics of North America is also published in Spanish by McGraw-Hill Interamericana Editores S. A., P.O. Box 5-237, 06500 Mexico, D.F., Mexico.

Medical Clinics of North America is covered in *MEDLINE/PubMed (Index Medicus), Current Contents, ASCA, Excerpta Medica, Science Citation Index,* and *ISI/BIOMED.*

PROGRAM OBJECTIVE
The goal of the *Medical Clinics of North America* is to keep practicing physicians up to date with current clinical practice by providing timely articles reviewing the state of the art in patient care.

TARGET AUDIENCE
All practicing physicians and other healthcare professionals.

LEARNING OBJECTIVES
Upon completion of this activity, participants will be able to:
1. Explain the pathology of cardiometabolic disorder(s) and its risk factors regarding age, race, gender, and special populations.
2. Discuss the identification and diagnosis of cardiometabolic disorders using the appropriate assessment, screening and diagnostic tools to mitigate the effects of cardiometabolic disorder(s) on specific patient populations and to develop strategies for disease management effectively.
3. Review the efficacy, risks, and benefits of treatment strategies, including lifestyle changes and pharmacotherapy.

ACCREDITATION
The Elsevier Office of Continuing Medical Education (EOCME) is accredited by the Accreditation Council for Continuing Medical Education (ACCME) to provide continuing medical education for physicians.

The EOCME designates this journal-based CME activity for a maximum of 13 *AMA PRA Category 1 Credit*(s)™. Physicians should claim only the credit commensurate with the extent of their participation in the activity.

All other healthcare professionals requesting continuing education credit for this enduring material will be issued a certificate of participation.

DISCLOSURE OF CONFLICTS OF INTEREST
The EOCME assesses conflict of interest with its instructors, faculty, planners, and other individuals who are in a position to control the content of CME activities. All relevant conflicts of interest that are identified are thoroughly vetted by EOCME for fair balance, scientific objectivity, and patient care recommendations. EOCME is committed to providing its learners with CME activities that promote improvements or quality in healthcare and not a specific proprietary business or a commercial interest.

The planning committee, staff, authors and editors listed below have identified no financial relationships or relationships to products or devices they or their spouse/life partner have with commercial interest related to the content of this CME activity:
Michael Parker Ayers, MD, FACC; Najdat Bazarbashi, MD; Jessica Chowns, CGC; Jordana B. Cohen, MD, MSCE; Andrew Gagel, MD; Samuel Gnanakumar; Aziz Hammoud, MD; Alvis Cole Headen, BS; Lily Hoffman-Andrews, CGC; Douglas S. Jacoby, MD; Howard M. Julien, MD, MPH, ML; Vivek T. Kulkarni, MD; Christopher Lee, MD; Juliette Kathleen Logan, MD; Amy Marzolf, CRNP; Christopher B. McFadden, MD; Reed Mszar, MPH; Paul Nona, MD; Cameron K. Ormiston, BS; Merlin Packiam; Nosheen Reza, MD; Ashley Rosander, BS; Cori Russell, MD; Liann Abu Salman, MD; Christeen Samuel; Monika Sanghavi, MD; Harini Sarathy, MBBS, MHS; Andrew Siaw-Asamoah, BA, MPhil; Pam R. Taub, MD, FACC; Doreen Thomas-Payne, MSN, BSN, RN, PMHNP-BC; Paul D. Thompson, MD; Jourdan Triebwasser, MD, MA; Gayley B. Webb, CRNP; Fawzi Zghyer, MD

The planning committee, staff, authors and editors listed below have identified financial relationships or relationships to products or devices they or their spouse/life partner have with commercial interest related to the content of this CME activity:
Zahid Ahmad, MD: *Consultant*: Akcea Therapeutics, Esperion

Douglas S. Jacoby, MD: *Consultant/Advisor:* AstraZeneca, Regeneron

Seth S. Martin, MD, MHS, FACC, FAHA, FASPC: *Research Support*: Apple, Google, Amgen Inc; *Consultant*: Akcea Therapeutics, Amgen, AstraZeneca, Esperion, Kaneka, Novo Nordisk, Quest Diagnostics, Regeneron, REGENXBIO, Sanofi, 89bio

Michael Miller, MD: *Advisor*: Amarin, Pfizer, 89bio

Anjali Tiku Owens, MD: *Consultant*: MyoKardia, Cytokinetics

Michael D. Shapiro, DO, MCR: *Advisor*: Amgen Inc, Esperion, Novartis

Daniel Soffer, MD: *Consultant*: Akcea Therapeutics, Novartis; *Research Support*: Amgen Inc, Astra-Zeneca, Ionis, Novartis, Regeneron, RegenXBio

UNAPPROVED/OFF-LABEL USE DISCLOSURE

The EOCME requires CME faculty to disclose to the participants;

1. When products or procedures being discussed are off-label, unlabelled, experimental, and/or investigational (not US Food and Drug Administration [FDA] approved); and
2. Any limitations on the information presented, such as data that are preliminary or that represent ongoing research, interim analyses, and/or unsupported opinions. Faculty may discuss information about pharmaceutical agents that is outside of FDA-approved labelling. This information is intended solely for CME and is not intended to promote off-label use of these medications. If you have any questions, contact the medical affairs department of the manufacturer for the most recent prescribing information.

TO ENROLL

To enroll in the *Medical Clinics of North America* Continuing Medical Education program, call customer service at 1-800-654-2452 or sign up online at http; //www.theclinics.com/home/cme. The CME program is available to subscribers for an additional annual fee of USD 324.00.

METHOD OF PARTICIPATION

In order to claim credit, participants must complete the following;

1. Complete enrolment as indicated above.
2. Read the activity.
3. Complete the CME Test and Evaluation. Participants must achieve a score of 70% on the test. All CME Tests and Evaluations must be completed online.

CME INQUIRIES/SPECIAL NEEDS

For all CME inquiries or special needs, please contact elsevierCME@elsevier.com.

MEDICAL CLINICS OF NORTH AMERICA

SERIES OF RELATED INTEREST

Primary Care: Clinics in Office Practice
Psychiatrics Clinic

Contributors

CONSULTING EDITOR

JACK ENDE, MD, MACP
The Schaeffer Professor of Medicine, Perelman School of Medicine, University of Pennsylvania, Philadelphia, Pennsylvania

EDITOR

DOUGLAS S. JACOBY, MD
Louis R Dinon, MD Teaching Chair of Clinical Cardiology, Chief of the Division of Cardiology, Pennsylvania Hospital, Medical Director, Penn Medicine Center for Preventive Cardiology and Lipid Management Professor of Clinical Medicine, University of Pennsylvania, Philadelphia, Pennsylvania

AUTHORS

ZAHID AHMAD, MD
Division of Nutrition and Metabolic Disease, Department of Internal Medicine, University of Texas Southwestern Medical Center, Dallas, Texas, USA

MICHAEL PARKER AYERS, MD, FACC
Assistant Professor, Division of Cardiovascular Medicine, University of Virginia, Heart and Vascular Center Fontaine, Charlottesville, Virginia

NAJDAT BAZARBASHI, MD
Department of Medicine, University of Maryland School of Medicine, Baltimore, Maryland

JESSICA CHOWNS, CGC
Division of Cardiovascular Medicine, Department of Medicine, Center for Inherited Cardiovascular Disease, Perelman School of Medicine, University of Pennsylvania, Perelman Center for Advanced Medicine, Philadelphia, Pennsylvania

JORDANA B. COHEN, MD, MSCE
Department of Biostatistics, Epidemiology, and Informatics, Renal-Electrolyte and Hypertension Division, Perelman School of Medicine, University of Pennsylvania, Philadelphia, Pennsylvania

ANDREW GAGEL, MD
Johns Hopkins School of Medicine, Baltimore, Maryland

AZIZ HAMMOUD, MD
Section of Cardiovascular Medicine, Department of Internal Medicine, Wake Forest University School of Medicine, Winston-Salem, North Carolina

ALVIS COLEMAN HEADEN, BS
Perelman School of Medicine, University of Pennsylvania, Philadelphia, Pennsylvania

LILY HOFFMAN-ANDREWS, CGC
Division of Cardiovascular Medicine, Department of Medicine, Center for Inherited Cardiovascular Disease, Perelman School of Medicine, University of Pennsylvania, Perelman Center for Advanced Medicine, Philadelphia, Pennsylvania

VIVEK T. KULKARNI, MD
Division of Cardiovascular Medicine, Department of Medicine, Perelman School of Medicine, University of Pennsylvania, Philadelphia, Pennsylvania, USA

HOWARD M. JULIEN, MD, MPH, ML
Assistant Professor of Clinical Medicine, Perelman School of Medicine, University of Pennsylvania, Philadelphia, Pennsylvania; Penn Cardiovascular Outcomes, Quality, and Evaluative Research Center, Penn Cardiovascular Center for Health Equity and Social Justice

CHRISTOPHER LEE, MD
Department of Medicine, Pennsylvania Hospital, University of Pennsylvania Health System, Philadelphia, Pennsylvania

JULIETTE KATHLEEN LOGAN, MD
Fellow, Division of Cardiovascular Medicine, University of Virginia, Heart and Vascular Center Fontaine, Charlottesville, Virginia

SETH S. MARTIN, MD, MHS, FACC, FAHA, FASPC
Johns Hopkins School of Medicine, Associate Professor of Medicine and Cardiology, Director, Advanced Lipid Disorders Program, Ciccarone Center for the Prevention of Cardiovascular Disease, Baltimore, Maryland

AMY MARZOLF, CRNP
Division of Cardiovascular Medicine, Department of Medicine, Center for Inherited Cardiovascular Disease, Perelman School of Medicine, University of Pennsylvania, Perelman Center for Advanced Medicine, Philadelphia, Pennsylvania

CHRISTOPHER B. McFADDEN, MD
Associate Professor, Department of Medicine, Cooper Medical School of Rowan University, Camden, New Jersey

MICHAEL MILLER, MD, FACC, FAHA
Professor, Department of Cardiovascular Medicine, University of Maryland School of Medicine, Baltimore, Maryland

REED MSZAR, MPH
Yale Center for Outcomes Research and Evaluation, New Haven, Connecticut, USA

PAUL NONA, MD
Fellow in Cardiovascular Disease, Department of Internal Medicine, Division of Cardiology, Detroit, Michigan

CAMERON K. ORMISTON, BS
Division of Cardiovascular Medicine, Department of Medicine, University of California, San Diego, San Diego, California

ANJALI TIKU OWENS, MD
Division of Cardiovascular Medicine, Department of Medicine, Center for Inherited Cardiovascular Disease, Perelman School of Medicine, University of Pennsylvania, Perelman Center for Advanced Medicine, Philadelphia, Pennsylvania

NOSHEEN REZA, MD
Division of Cardiovascular Medicine, Department of Medicine, Center for Inherited Cardiovascular Disease, Perelman School of Medicine, University of Pennsylvania, Perelman Center for Advanced Medicine, Philadelphia, Pennsylvania

ASHLEY ROSANDER, BS
Division of Cardiovascular Medicine, Department of Medicine, University of California, San Diego, San Diego, California

CORI RUSSELL, MD
Senior Staff Cardiologist, Department of Internal Medicine, Division of Cardiology, Detroit, Michigan

LIANN ABU SALMAN, MD
Renal-Electrolyte and Hypertension Division, Renal Division, Perelman School of Medicine, University of Pennsylvania, Hospital of the University of Pennsylvania, Philadelphia, Pennsylvania

CHRISTEEN SAMUEL
Johns Hopkins School of Medicine, Baltimore, Maryland

MONIKA SANGHAVI, MD
Associate Professor of Medicine, Division of Cardiology, University of Pennsylvania, Philadelphia, Pennsylvania

HARINI SARATHY, MBBS, MHS
Division of Nephrology and Hypertension, Zuckerberg San Francisco General Hospital, University of California, San Francisco, San Francisco, California

MICHAEL D. SHAPIRO, DO, MCR
Fred M. Parrish Professor of Cardiology and Molecular Medicine, Section of Cardiovascular Medicine, Department of Internal Medicine, Wake Forest University School of Medicine, Center for Prevention of Cardiovascular Disease, Winston-Salem, North Carolina

DANIEL SOFFER, MD
Division of Cardiovascular Medicine, Department of Medicine, Perelman School of Medicine, University of Pennsylvania, Philadelphia, Pennsylvania, USA

ANDREW SIAW-ASAMOAH, BA, MPhil
Perelman School of Medicine, University of Pennsylvania, Philadelphia, Pennsylvania

PAM R. TAUB, MD, FACC
Division of Cardiovascular Medicine, Department of Medicine, University of California, San Diego, California

PAUL D. THOMPSON, MD
Chief of Cardiology – Emeritus, Hartford Hospital, Hartford, Connecticut; Professor of Medicine, University of Connecticut

JOURDAN E. TRIEBWASSER, MD, MA
Assistant Professor of Obstetrics and Gynecology, Division of Maternal-Fetal Medicine, University of University of Michigan, Ann Arbor, Michigan

GAYLEY B. WEBB, CRNP
Division of Cardiovascular Medicine, Department of Medicine, Perelman School of
Medicine, University of Pennsylvania, Philadelphia, Pennsylvania, USA

FAWZI ZGHYER, MD
Johns Hopkins School of Medicine, Baltimore, Maryland

Contents

 Video content accompanies this article at http://www.medical. theclinics.com.

> This review highlights the key components of a heart-healthy diet and pre-
> sents an evidence-based overview of recent research. Diets that increase
> plant-based food sources and healthy unsaturated fats consumption and
> limit foods that are processed and/or high in sodium, refined sugar, and
> saturated fat are recommended. Dietary modification can be supple-
> mented with lifestyle-based therapies (eg, exercise, time-restricted eating)
> to maximize clinical benefit and achieve the "cardiometabolic jackpot."
> Physicians should take into account cultural preferences, affordability
> and accessibility of foods, and their patients' cultural values or expecta-
> tions when recommending dietary interventions.

> The cardiovascular epidemiologist, Jeremy Morris, called physical activity
> "the best bargain in public health," but few clinicians use exercise and
> physical activity in their practice. Clinicians should routinely inquire about
> physical activity and recommend that patients achieve the minimal levels
> recommended by the 2018 Physical Activity Guidelines for Americans.
> Clinician should avoid unnecessary testing that discourages patients
> from an active lifestyle. Patients after myocardial infarction, cardiac sur-
> gery, or the diagnosis of heart failure or claudication should be referred
> to an exercise-based cardiac rehab program. Physical activity and exer-
> cise training may be a clinical bargain, but as with all medical interventions,
> it must be used to be effective.

> The treatment of elevated blood pressure (BP) can improve cardiovascular
> (CV) event rates. Current BP targets depend on expected CV event rates in
> individuals as assessed by concurrent medical conditions and other risk
> factors. Importantly, the means by which BP is measured has evolved.
> This evolution is driven by recognition that techniques different than

routine office BP measurements can provide a better assessment of future CV risk.

Hypertension is a major cause of cardiovascular morbidity and mortality globally. Many patients with hypertension have secondary causes of hypertension that merit further evaluation. For example, secondary hypertension can result in target organ damage to the heart, kidneys, and brain independent of the effects of blood pressure. Several causes benefit from targeted therapies to supplement first-line antihypertensive agents. However, secondary hypertension is often underrecognized. The goal of this review is to highlight optimal approaches to the diagnosis and management of common causes of secondary hypertension, including primary aldosteronism, renovascular hypertension, obstructive sleep apnea, and drug-induced hypertension.

One's total atherosclerotic plaque burden is related to his or her cumulative exposure to low-density lipoprotein cholesterol (LDL-C) and other apoB-containing lipoproteins. Long-term exposure to lower LDL-C levels is associated with a lower risk of cardiovascular events compared with shorter term exposure to lower LDL-C. New lipid-reducing agents have been able to reduce LDL-C to previously unseen levels, showing efficacy in safely decreasing rates of atherosclerotic cardiovascular disease in primary and secondary prevention populations. To date, an LDL-C level below which there is no clinical benefit has not yet been identified.

Hypertriglyceridemia (HTG) is among the most common dyslipidemias seen in clinical practice. Studies in recent years have demonstrated a causal relationship between triglyceride-rich lipoproteins (TRL) and cardiovascular disease (CVD). This is primarily due to enhanced atherogenicity of cholesterol-enriched remnants, the metabolic byproducts of TRLs. While desirable TGs are less than 150 mg/dL (fasting) or 175 mg/dL (nonfasting), optimal levels are likely to be less than 100 mg/dL. First line treatment for HTG is directed at lifestyle and includes weight loss. National guidelines recommend that adults aged 40-75 years with elevated triglycerides (175-499 mg/dL) and increased CVD risk (i.e., 7.5% or higher) have statins initiated or intensified after lifestyle and secondary factors are addressed. The recent results of the REDUCE-IT study also support consideration of Icosapent ethyl, the highly purified EPA, to further reduce CVD risk in high-risk patients with HTG.

Many cardiovascular disorders have underlying genetic causes. Clinical genetic testing for cardiovascular disease has become widely available and can be useful for diagnosis, management, and cascade screening in selected conditions and circumstances. This article gives an overview of the current state of genetic testing in inherited cardiovascular conditions, who can benefit from it, and the associated challenges.

Genetic lipid disorders, ranging from common dyslipidemias such as familial hypercholesterolemia, lipoprotein (a), and familial combined hyperlipidemia to rare disorders including familial chylomicronemia syndrome and inherited hypoalphalipoproteinemias (ie, Tangier and fish eye diseases), affect millions of individuals in the United States and tens of millions around the world and are often undiagnosed in the general population. Clinicians should take into consideration the potential of inherited lipid disorders or syndromes when severe derangements in lipid parameters are observed. Patients' combined genotype and phenotype should be evaluated in conjunction with a host of environmental factors impacting their risk of atherosclerotic cardiovascular disease.Genetic lipid disorders, ranging from common dyslipidemias such as familial hypercholesterolemia, lipoprotein (a), and familial combined hyperlipidemia to rare disorders including familial chylomicronemia syndrome and inherited hypoalphalipoproteinemias (ie, Tangier and fish eye diseases), affect millions of individuals in the United States and tens of millions around the world and are often undiagnosed in the general population. Clinicians should take into consideration the potential of inherited lipid disorders or syndromes when severe derangements in lipid parameters are observed. Patients' combined genotype and phenotype should be evaluated in conjunction with a host of environmental factors impacting their risk of atherosclerotic cardiovascular disease.

Inflammation plays a well-established role in the development and progression of atherosclerosis. Individuals exposed to chronic inflammation are at an increased risk of developing cardiovascular disease, including coronary artery disease and heart failure, independent of associated traditional risk factors. Traditional risk assessment tools and calculators underestimate the true cardiac risk in this population. In addition to this, there is a lack of awareness on the association between inflammation and cardiovascular disease. These factors lead to undertreatment in terms of preventive cardiac care in patients with chronic inflammatory disease.

Foreword
In Evidence We Trust

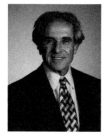

Jack Ende, MD, MACP
Consulting Editor

Select antibiotic treatment for a patient with pneumonia and watch him get better, or not. Initiate anti-inflammatory medication for a patient with a swollen great toe, and you will know straight away if he has gout. Begin prophylactic migraine medication for a patient with recurrent headaches, and if she responds, you can surmise that you have done her some good. Primary care practice is filled with such examples, where physicians can initiate an intervention and determine, often very quickly, whether the intervention is worthwhile.

But what about when we set out not to treat a disease that we know the patient has, but, rather, to prevent a disease that the patient may or may not develop? That, dear colleagues, is why prevention is so challenging. We just cannot be sure if we are doing the patient any good. Yes, of course, we can observe the LDL-cholesterol go down, or the blood pressure reach a target range. But lipids and blood pressure readings are intermediate outcomes, not necessarily clinical outcomes.

Yet what can be more important in the practice of medicine than preventing a myocardial infarction or stroke, or forestalling heart failure or peripheral arterial disease? Are not health promotion and disease prevention among our field's most important goals?

In the end, therefore, in developing strategies for preventing morbidity and decreasing rates of mortality, clinicians must base their decisions upon the best-quality evidence. This is no more essential than in preventive cardiology. When we recommend that our patients modify their diet, exercise, take medications, and undergo screening procedures, we owe it to them to base these recommendations on high-quality evidence that supports important clinical outcomes. No practitioner can amass this evidence from his or her own practice. Rather, we must rely on published data and bias-free guidance, assembled by experts. That is what readers of this issue of *Medical Clinics of North America* will find in "Update in Preventive Cardiology." Guest Editor, Douglas S. Jacoby, has, first, identified the most important topics relevant to clinical

Med Clin N Am 106 (2022) xv–xvi
https://doi.org/10.1016/j.mcna.2021.11.014
0025-7125/22/© 2021 Published by Elsevier Inc.

practice; then he has assembled teams of experts to deliver evidence-based guidance that clinicians can deploy on behalf of their patient. We can trust this guidance, just as we trust our clinical observations.

Jack Ende, MD, MACP
The Schaeffer Professor of Medicine
Perelman School of Medicine
The University of Pennsylvania
Philadelphia, PA 19104, USA

E-mail address:
jack.ende@pennmedicine.upenn.edu

Preface

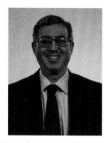

Douglas S. Jacoby, MD
Editor

Cardiovascular disease is the leading cause of death worldwide, and the number of people dying from cardiovascular disease is continuing to rise. This enormous burden of disease gradually develops during one's lifetime from both genetic risk and modifiable risk, making it an ideal target for prevention.

Understanding genetic risk helps identify at-risk individuals and their families earlier, to change the natural history of disease. Similarly, by addressing the modifiable risk, it is possible to substantially decrease the burden of cardiovascular disease. Lifestyle and pharmacologic interventions can reduce cardiovascular events by more than 75%, which would save millions of lives every year.

The modifiable risk factors with the greatest impact on the burden of cardiovascular disease include elevated blood pressure, poor diet, and elevated LDL cholesterol. In this issue of *Medical Clinics of North America*, talented authors address these modifiable risk factors and many others. There is advice from leading professionals to help readers gain insight into heart-healthy lifestyle choices, diagnosis and control of risk factors, and cutting-edge strategies to understand and reduce cardiovascular risk. Beyond these risk factors, they address other important areas within preventive cardiology, such as exercise, triglyceride management, assessing cardiovascular risk, inflammation, women's cardiovascular health, drug interactions, and health disparities.

Preventive cardiology as a field has grown substantially in breadth and depth over the last decade. Genetic knowledge has exploded. The importance of lifestyle has gained significant traction. Many new classes of safe medications have shown cardiovascular benefit in treating cholesterol and other metabolic risk factors. A multitude of national and international organizations now targets different aspects of disease.

Med Clin N Am 106 (2022) xvii–xviii
https://doi.org/10.1016/j.mcna.2021.11.015
0025-7125/22/© 2021 Published by Elsevier Inc.

This issue, focusing on preventive cardiology, provides key updates in this rapidly expanding field. If reading this saves even one life, the mission has been accomplished, though it is hoped it will save many, many more.

Douglas S. Jacoby, MD
Department of Medicine
University of Pennsylvania
Philadelphia, PA 19106, USA

E-mail address:
Douglas.Jacoby@pennmedicine.upenn.edu

Heart-Healthy Diets and the Cardiometabolic Jackpot

Cameron K. Ormiston, BS, Ashley Rosander, BS, Pam R. Taub, MD*

KEYWORDS

- Plant-based diet • Cardiovascular disease • Nutrition • Cultural competency
- Obesity

KEY POINTS

- The key elements of a heart-healthy diet are a variety of vegetables, fruits, whole grains, low-fat or fat-free dairy, plant-based protein sources, and unsaturated oils. Saturated fats, red meat, and added sugars should be reduced and replaced by healthier alternatives.
- The "cardiometabolic jackpot" involves supplementing nutritional intervention with lifestyle changes, such as exercise or time-restricted eating (having a daily eating window of 8–10 hours), maximizing the benefits of healthy eating.
- Among popular diets currently available, the Mediterranean diet and Ornish diet have the strongest evidence supporting their clinical use.
- A patient's sociocultural and socioeconomic context must be considered when implementing dietary or lifestyle interventions. This includes cultural food practices, affordable and accessible foods, and cultural values or expectations.

 Video content accompanies this article at http://www.medical.theclinics.com.

INTRODUCTION

The increasing rate of cardiovascular disease (CVD) is intricately linked with diet and lifestyle, although health care providers are often poorly educated on evidence-based lifestyle interventions. Given both medical students and physicians report receiving inadequate training in nutrition education and more than 25% of primary care visits are nutrition-related, the need to address this knowledge gap is becoming increasingly important.[1,2]

Unfortunately, foods high in sodium, saturated fat (SF), added sugar, and processed foods are on the rise because of globalization, convenience, affordability, and widespread popularity and marketing. Consequently, US CVD rates have increased by 25% since 1990 and greater than 66% of Americans are overweight or obese.[3,4]

Division of Cardiovascular Medicine, UC San Diego, 9500 Gilman Drive MC 7411, La Jolla, San Diego, CA 92037-7411, USA
* Corresponding author. Division of Cardiovascular Medicine, University of California San Diego, 9300 Campus Point Drive, Mail Code #7414, La Jolla, CA 92037.
E-mail address: ptaub@health.ucsd.edu

Med Clin N Am 106 (2022) 235–247
https://doi.org/10.1016/j.mcna.2021.11.001
0025-7125/22/© 2021 Elsevier Inc. All rights reserved.

Obesity is a gateway to chronic disease conditions, such as metabolic syndrome, hyperlipidemia, type 2 diabetes (T2D), and hypertension, which all confer increased risk of CVD. Moreover, obesity disproportionately impacts ethnic and racial minorities, with African American and Hispanic/Latino adults having double the risk of developing obesity compared to White Americans.[5] These disparities are due to inequitable access to economic, educational, and health resources, where racial and ethnic minorities experience significantly greater socioeconomic, structural, and environmental barriers to health.[6]

To address the increase of CVD and obesity, the American Heart Association (AHA) issued diet guidelines arguing for the increased consumption of fruits, vegetables, fish, and fiber, and the cutting down on foods that are processed and/or high in sodium, cholesterol, and SF.[7] This review focuses on the key elements of a heart-healthy diet, popular diets and their strengths and limitations, the cardiometabolic jackpot, and special considerations for nutritional counseling.

DISCUSSION: HEART-HEALTHY DIET GUIDELINES

A diet focused on nutrient-rich foods from a variety of natural sources is the foundation of health optimization and CVD risk reduction, reducing myocardial infarction (MI) risk by 17% to 23%.[8] A healthy diet includes a moderate consumption of a variety of colorful vegetables, legumes, fruits, whole grains, low-fat or fat-free dairy, plant-based protein sources, and unsaturated oils (**Table 1**). SF and added sugars should be less than 10% of one's total daily caloric intake, and sodium consumption should be < 2300 mg/d[7] Alarmingly, people who acquire $\geq$25% of their calories from sugar have double the risk of CVD mortality compared with those who have sugar comprising less than 10% of their diet (P = .004).[9] Although advertised as sugar-free and healthier, diet soda is associated with increased risk of metabolic syndrome and T2D, possibly because of

Table 1
Best foods to consume and avoid

Consume Most of the Time	Consume Occasionally	Avoid
Whole fruits and raw vegetables (citrus fruits, apples, pears, and berries; allium, carrots, cruciferous, and leafy greens)	Roasted/salted nuts	Highly processed foods
Fish and lean meats (salmon, poultry)	Moderate alcohol consumption	Foods with added sugars
Legumes	Fruit and vegetable juices can be high in calories and sugar, but low in fiber	Artificial sweeteners
Raw nuts		High sodium foods
Low sodium and no added sugar options		Excess alcohol
Fortified foods (eg, whole-grain cereals)		Oils or fats that are solid at room temperature (coconut oil, margarine)
Foods that fit the Mediterranean or other plant-based diets		

artificial sweeteners increasing the risk of insulin resistance due to the pancreas equating the sweeteners as glucose, triggering an insulin response.[10] Also, every 1000 mg of dietary sodium intake is linked to a 6% increase in CVD risk.[11]

Legumes, plant-based proteins, and fish are excellent protein sources and preferable to red meat because chronic red meat consumption increases the risk of adverse cardiovascular events and mortality.[12] Legumes and plant-based sources are nutritious and cardioprotective substitutes for meat-based protein sources. In fact, having 1 daily serving of legumes (130 g) significantly decreases low-density lipoprotein (LDL) levels compared with no legume consumption.[13] Legumes are high in antioxidants, fiber, and nutrients, very low in SF, and are cholesterol free.[14] Legume protein content is on par with red meat, containing 20% to 45% protein, whereas lean red meat contains 26% to 27%.[15] Legumes can also play a key role in preventing CVD, cancers, and other degenerative diseases, with Bazzano and colleagues[16] showing legume consumption significantly decreases the incidence of coronary heart disease (CHD) ($P = .002$) and CVD ($P = .02$). Furthermore, Kelemen and colleagues[17] showed replacing animal proteins with plant-based proteins can decrease CHD events by 30% ($P = .02$). When comparing legume consumption ≥ 4 times per week to <1 time per week, eating legumes lowered CHD and CVD risk by 22% and 11%, respectively.[16] Legumes can also aid in weight loss, with 1 daily serving of legumes significantly decreasing body weight compared with diets without legumes, even when adhering to noncaloric restriction diets ($P = .03$).[18] One concern of having solely plant-based protein sources, however, is the risk of becoming deficient in essential micronutrients, such as vitamin B12, which can be prevented through supplementation.[19]

Fruit and vegetables are essential, universal components of a heart-healthy diet. Total fruit and vegetable consumption has an inverse relationship with CVD, CHD, and stroke incidence.[20] Three to 4 daily servings of fruits and vegetables (375–500 g) can significantly reduce all-cause mortality and improve cardiovascular health. Among fruits, citrus, apples, pears, and berries exhibit the most cardiovascular benefits; allium, carrots, cruciferous, and leafy greens are the most beneficial among vegetables.[20] Fruits and vegetables have a benefits threshold, however, with CVD risk and mortality being inversely related to combined fruit and vegetable consumption until 800 g/d, after which no benefits are observed.[21] Raw vegetables are more strongly associated with lower mortality, cancer, and CVD risk than cooked vegetables, possibly because of degradation and loss of nutrients during the cooking process.[21]

Substituting high-glycemic carbohydrates and refined grains with complex and low-glycemic carbohydrates can reduce all-cause mortality, CVD, and cancer risk.[22,23] In fact, 1 to 2 daily servings (16–32 g) of whole grains and fibrous foods, which contain phytonutrients and germ layers that are absent in refined grains, decreases CVD risk by 10% to 20%.[22] Current AHA guidelines suggest eating 6 servings of grain per day (≥ 3 of which should be whole grain).[24]

Comparing fiber types, viscous fiber (fruits, beans, oats) and cereal grains are more cardioprotective than insoluble fiber (whole wheat). Although high-glycemic foods' exacerbation of CVD risk is well known, the benefits of low-glycemic foods have come under recent scrutiny. For example, Sacks and colleagues[25] showed low-glycemic foods had minimal effects on insulin sensitivity, blood pressure (BP), triglyceride, and cholesterol levels. Fiber content is therefore a more reliable measure of cardiovascular benefits.[26]

Dietary fats are generally classified as unsaturated, saturated, or trans fats. Higher consumption of trans fats is positively correlated with lipid risk factors for CVD, raising

CHD risk and mortality by 21% and 28%, respectively.[27] Trans fats and SF should be substituted with unsaturated fat (polyunsaturated is preferred), complex carbohydrates/whole grains, and protein. Meta-analyses show every 5% of energy from SF replaced with an isocaloric amount of polyunsaturated fats can reduce CHD events and risk by 10% and 27%, respectively.[23,28] Moreover, decreasing SF consumption can improve lipid profiles.[29] Fish, particularly fatty fish like salmon, are excellent sources of protein and omega-3 polyunsaturated fatty acids, significantly lowering BP and mortality.[30] In the Diet and Reinfarction trial (n = 2033), higher fish consumption was linked to a 29% reduction in total mortality and 32% reduction in CHD mortality compared with increased intake of grains or decreased total fat.[31] In addition, replacing SF with whole grains can reduce CHD risk by 6%.[32]

Although typically high in SF, dairy products can have a positive impact on CVD risk or diabetes, regardless of fat content. The PURE study (n = 135,335) showed greater than 2 daily servings of dairy is inversely correlated with mortality, major CVD, and stroke when compared with no dairy consumption.[33] Compared with unsaturated fat, however, dairy fat significantly increases LDL and total cholesterol levels ($P > .05$).[34] Current literature and guidelines therefore suggest limiting SF intake and replacing it with polyunsaturated fats and complex carbohydrates.

CURRENT EVIDENCE ON POPULAR DIETS

Several diets have recently emerged as popular in the health care field and mainstream media. Each diet's key components, current evidence, and utility for cardiovascular risk reduction are discussed below (**Table 2**).

Mediterranean Diet

Named for its regional and historical roots, the Mediterranean diet (MD) consists of high consumption of whole grains and cereal, legumes, fruits, and vegetables as well as moderate consumption of dairy products and alcohol. It is also characterized by low consumption of meat and meat products, although fish is often a source of protein.[35]

The MD has some of the strongest evidence for CVD prevention.[29] Many trials and critical reviews have validated the health effects of this diet, showing that it reduces CHD, ischemic stroke, and total CVD.[35–37] In fact, MD adherence is associated with a 40% CVD risk reduction.[38] In the Lyon Diet Heart study (n = 423), post-MI participants who were randomized to the MD group experienced protective effects of the lifestyle change even 4 years after the MI and had significantly lower incidence of recurrent MI compared with the Western diet group ($P = 0.0001$).[39] In addition, the degree of MD adherence has been shown to have an inverse relationship with total mortality, and cardiovascular and MI incidence and mortality.[40]

As a result of strong evidence supporting this dietary lifestyle, major societies recommend the MD to address multiple comorbidities, including hyperlipidemia (recommended by AHA), T2D (recommended by ADA), and obesity (recommended by the American Association of Clinical Endocrinology).[29]

Ornish Diet

The Ornish diet is vegetarian and consists of 10% fat, complex carbohydrates, and whole foods while discouraging simple sugars.[41]

The LIFESTYLE Heart Trial (n = 35) examined the difference in coronary atherosclerosis progression and cardiac event incidence in a control group versus an "Ornish" intensive lifestyle change, which includes dietary intervention, aerobic exercise, stress

Table 2
Key components of the Mediterranean, Ornish, Pritikin, ketogenic, and paleolithic diet

Diet	Components of Diet	Key Studies	Long-Term Adherence
Mediterranean	High consumption: whole-grains and cereal, legumes, fruits, and vegetables Moderate consumption: dairy products and alcohol. Low consumption: meat and meat products	Lyon Diet Heart study (n = 204 control, n = 219 experimental)[39] PREDIMED study (n = 7447)[51]	Lyon Diet Heart study: most intervention patients were still closely adhering to the Mediterranean diet several years after randomization PREDIMED: Mediterranean diet group adherence scores were significantly higher than the control group 6 y after study completion (P < .0001); patients maintained sufficient adherence to the Mediterranean diet after 6 y
Ornish	Vegetarian, 10% fat, complex carbohydrates, and whole foods. Discourages simple sugars	LIFESTYLE Heart Trial (n = 35)[41]	LIFESTYLE Heart Trial: 100% compliance after 5 y
Pritikin	Whole foods, whole-grains, fruits, vegetables, and lean meats, such as fish and poultry. Low fat	"Effect of short-term Pritikin diet therapy on the metabolic syndrome" (n = 67)[52]	80% of patients reported dietary compliance after 5 y; however, more trials are needed[52,53]
Ketogenic	Low consumption of carbohydrates and a high ingestion of fats, including saturated fats	"Effect of a plant-based, low-fat diet vs an animal-based, ketogenic diet on ad libitum energy intake" (n = 20)[47]	Unlikely to be sustained beyond 1–2 y[54]
Paleolithic	Meat, fruits, vegetables. No dairy or grains	"Effects of a short-term intervention with a paleolithic diet in healthy volunteers" (n = 14)[49]	80% compliance in 29 male patients with ischemic heart disease after 12 wk[55] Trials still needed for long-term assessment

management coaching, smoking cessation, and psychosocial support groups. After 5 years, the Ornish group experienced coronary atherosclerosis regression, whereas the control group experienced progression and more cardiac event incidence.[41] In a 1-year randomized trial of 4 popular diets in which diet was the only intervention, the Ornish diet (n = 40) exhibited an ~10% reduction in the high-density lipoprotein (HDL)/LDL ratio and reduced body weight, insulin, total cholesterol/HDL ratio, and inflammation.[42]

Pritikin Diet

The Pritikin diet consists of whole foods, whole grains, fruits, vegetables, and lean meats, such as fish and poultry.[43] This diet limits calorically dense, high-fat foods, which leads to a reduced total caloric and cholesterol intake.[43] Therefore, the Pritikin diet is used as a low-fat diet to promote weight loss and overall cardiovascular health.

Ketogenic Diet

Although this diet has proven to be popular for weight loss in the past decade, there are precautions that patients should take note of before starting this diet.

The ketogenic diet consists of a very low consumption of carbohydrates and a high ingestion of fats, including SF.[44] In cancer treatment, the ketogenic diet can sensitize cancer cells to treatment by creating an unfavorable metabolic environment.[45] This diet has also exhibited both positive and negative effects on the gut microbiota.[46]

In a randomized controlled trial (n = 20) in which the ketogenic diet was tested against a low-fat plant-based diet, the ketogenic diet resulted in significantly more caloric intake ($P < .0001$).[47] Although the ketogenic diet may lead to short-term weight loss, it also raises LDL-cholesterol and can lead to hyperlipidemia, which has long-term cardiovascular consequences.[44]

Paleolithic Diet

The paleolithic, or "paleo" diet, has been controversially advertised by non–health experts as a "cure-all" for various diseases. This diet stems from the idea that modern life is not in tune with our ancestral human metabolism and people should only eat what cave people ate. This means meat, fruits, and vegetables, but no farm-born foods, such as grains and dairy products.[48]

In individuals with ischemic heart disease, the paleo diet decreased waist circumference (WC) and increased sensitivity to glucose.[48] In a 3-week pilot study (n = 14), paleo diet adherence significantly decreased body weight ($P < .001$), WC ($P = .001$), and systolic blood pressure (SBP; $P = .03$).[49] However, it should be noted that calcium consumption significantly decreased compared with prestudy consumption levels.

Some of the validity of the paleo diet stems from its focus on whole foods, leading to the benefits of avoiding the processed and artificial foods that plague the western menu. High glucose-containing foods found on the market today are avoided altogether, helping combat insulin resistance.[48] Although there is convincing evidence for short-term use of the paleo diet, long-term trials with varying patient populations are still needed.[50]

THE CARDIOMETABOLIC JACKPOT

A lifestyle-based approach using exercise and one's circadian rhythm can maximize the benefits of a heart-healthy diet (Video 1). Compared with diet-alone (D) and exercise-alone (E) interventions, exercise plus diet (E + D) produces the most changes in body composition.[56] In a study on 1-year D, E, and E + D interventions, the E + D arm exhibited significantly greater reductions in weight ($P_{D + E vs D} = 0.03$; $P_{D + E vs E} < 0.0001$), percent body fat ($P_{D + E vs D} = 0.005$; $P_{D + E vs E} < 0.0001$), and WC ($P_{D + E vs D} = 0.004$; $P_{D + E vs E} < 0.0001$).[57] Moreover, resistance training reduces more fat mass compared with endurance training and retains fat free mass.[56]

Time-restricted eating (TRE) is when one constricts all their caloric intake to a daily 8- to 10-hour eating window. A consistent feeding-fasting cycle facilitates circadian alignment, promoting metabolic and physiologic homeostasis.[58] This is crucial, as erratic or prolonged eating patterns increase the risk of CVD, insulin resistance, and obesity.[58] TRE has been shown to be effective in patients who are overweight/obese and in patients with metabolic syndrome, reducing insulin resistance, oxidative stress, WC, body fat %, and improving HbA_{1c}, BP, LDL, and non-HDL-cholesterol.[58] Moreover, TRE is more effective and easier to sustain than calorie counting or restriction.[59]

Early findings on combining TRE and exercise are promising. Comparing a 16:8 alternating TRE schedule with non-TRE while performing resistance training, Moro and colleagues[60] reported similar increases in muscle mass in both groups. However, the TRE group showed a greater reduction in fat mass and total body mass ($P = .04$), and improvements in glucose, HDL, and triglycerides.

SPECIAL CONSIDERATIONS
Low Socioeconomic Status

Even though plant-based diets are the most beneficial to cardiovascular health, they are not always accessible to everyone, particularly communities of low socioeconomic status (SES), which are disproportionately comprised of racial/ethnic minorities. Patients of low SES often cite food costs and a lack of knowledge about measuring or incorporating foods into their diet as significant barriers to prescribed diets.[61] Clinicians should therefore discuss with their patients the socioeconomic (eg, low-income, family responsibilities) or geographic barriers (eg, food deserts) they may face and tailor clinical guidance accordingly. For example, legumes, poultry, oils, nuts, milk, eggs, and whole-grain cereals are foods with ideal ratios of nutrition to price (**Fig. 1**).[62]

The use of smartphone applications to promote physical activity, health access, and community engagement has also shown promise in decreasing CVD disparities for

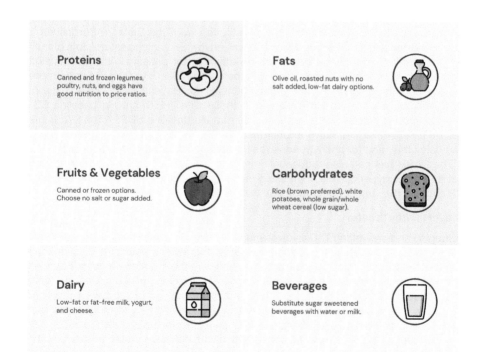

Proteins
Canned and frozen legumes, poultry, nuts, and eggs have good nutrition to price ratios.

Fats
Olive oil, roasted nuts with no salt added, low-fat dairy options.

Fruits & Vegetables
Canned or frozen options. Choose no salt or sugar added.

Carbohydrates
Rice (brown preferred), white potatoes, whole grain/whole wheat cereal (low sugar).

Dairy
Low-fat or fat-free milk, yogurt, and cheese.

Beverages
Substitute sugar sweetened beverages with water or milk.

Fig. 1. Heart-healthy diet on a budget. A guide for more affordable healthy food options.

minority populations.[63] Improving health literacy, physician and patient nutritional education, and access to resources and affordable foods is imperative to ameliorating barriers to health.

Cultural Competency

Given greater than 50% of the US population will be composed of individuals from different cultural backgrounds by 2050, practitioner knowledge of cultural food practices is essential to personalizing care to the patient.[64] Foods can have different roles and impacts on health across different cultures. For example, white rice is often cautioned against in some diets but holds symbolic and physical significance in some cultures; rice is a staple of many East Asian diets and is seen as vital and healthful. Moreover, clinicians should be aware of their patient's sociocultural role. For example, women with T2D may place the needs of others over their own and may not make family meals diabetes-friendly due to cultural expectations.[65]

Culture can also guide how one views foods and their nutritional quality. In traditional Chinese medicine, foods can be classified as "hot" or "cold," and one must eat a balance of hot and cold foods to maintain internal harmony or health.[61] Navajo tribes also have binary food classifications, categorizing them as "strong" or "filler" foods. Strong foods (eg, mutton, stew) promote health and are therapeutic and essential parts of religious ceremonies. Filler foods (eg. cheese, refined flour, and canned meat) are eaten daily.[61] Prescribed diets that suggest decreasing or discontinuing the consumption of these culturally valued foods may conflict with food practices and lifestyles. Practitioners should be mindful of possible conflicts between dietary counseling and the patient's sociocultural needs and adapt the care plan to those needs.

Patients with Hypertension

Combining reduced sodium intake (2-g restriction) with the Dietary Approaches to Stop Hypertension (DASH) diet, which focuses on low SF and cholesterol, lots of fruits and vegetables, and low-fat dairy, can be effective for patients with hypertension, significantly lowering SBP compared with the control diet ($P < .001$).[66] Furthermore, the low-sodium DASH diet has greater benefits for patients with higher baseline SBP, yielding a -11-mm Hg reduction in those with ≥ 150 mm Hg baseline SBP and -4 mm Hg in those with less than 130 mm Hg baseline SBP.[66] The DASH diet can be an effective alternative to pharmacotherapy for patients with hypertension or can delay the need for antihypertensives for patients at risk for hypertension.[67]

The DASH diet can also reduce inflammation and LDL-cholesterol.[68] For patients not at risk for hyperkalemia, increasing dietary potassium intake can also decrease BP and has the largest effect for those with higher baseline BP.[29]

Patients with Diabetes

Managing and preventing T2D involves much of the same guidelines described above. The American Diabetes Association has also suggested restricting carbohydrate intake to ~40% of total calories and focusing on whole grains, fruits, vegetables, and low-fat milk as one's carbohydrate sources. In addition, refined grains and foods with added sugar should be replaced by complex carbohydrate and low-glycemic alternatives. Sugar-sweetened beverage consumption should also be reduced, as each daily serving confers a 20% increase in T2D risk.[29] Trans fats can also increase T2D risk, and replacing 2% of trans fat consumption with polyunsaturated fats can reduce risk by 40%.[69] Lifestyle changes, such as increasing physical activity, should also be encouraged.

SUMMARY

To address the increase of CVD and obesity, clinicians should promote increased consumption of fruits, vegetables, fish, and foods high in fiber, and decreased consumption of foods that are processed and/or high in sugar, sodium, cholesterol, and SF. Combining a heart-healthy diet with synergistic lifestyle modification strategies, such as increased physical activity or TRE, can further optimize health, improving health outcomes. Special considerations should be made for patients of diverse backgrounds, patients of low SES, and patients with hypertension or diabetes, tailoring the diet intervention to their unique needs.

CLINICS CARE POINTS

- The Mediterranean diet and Ornish diet have the strongest evidence showing their effectiveness in lowering cardiovascular disease risk and mortality.
- Clinicians should be aware of other diets to educate their patients to follow them safely. For example, the ketogenic diet can easily be misconstrued and potentially lead to negative cardiovascular outcomes.
- Plant-based diets may run the risk of vitamin B12 deficiency because it is typically found in animal products. Supplementation may be necessary.
- To maximize the benefits of a healthy diet, lifestyle therapies, such as exercise, should also be implemented.
- Socioeconomic status and geographic region can be barriers to a patient's ability to adhere to dietary intervention, and clinicians should be aware of the barriers their patients face while giving nutritional advice.

DISCLOSURES

PRT: Amgen (consultant), Novo-Nordisk (consultant), Sanofi (consultant), Boehringer-Ingelheim (consultant), Epirium Bio (shareholder), Esperion therapeutics (consultant). CKO and AR have no disclosures to report. No funding was received in the writing of this manuscript.

SUPPLEMENTARY DATA

Supplementary data related to this article can be found online at https://doi.org/10.1016/j.mcna.2021.11.001.

REFERENCES

1. Kolasa KM, Rickett K. Barriers to providing nutrition counseling cited by physicians: a survey of primary care practitioners. Nutr Clin Pract 2010;25(5):502–9.
2. Devries S, Freeman AM. Nutrition education for cardiologists: the time has come. Curr Cardiol Rep 2017;19(9):77.
3. Products - data briefs - number 360 - February 2020. 2020. Available at: https://www.cdc.gov/nchs/products/databriefs/db360.htm. Accessed January 11, 2021.
4. Roth GA, Forouzanfar MH, Moran AE, et al. Demographic and epidemiologic drivers of global cardiovascular mortality. N Engl J Med 2015;372(14):1333–41.
5. Wang L, Southerland J, Wang K, et al. Ethnic differences in risk factors for obesity among adults in California, the United States. J Obes 2017;2017:2427483.

6. Petersen R, Pan L, Blanck HM. Racial and ethnic disparities in adult obesity in the United States: CDC's tracking to inform state and local action. Prev Chronic Dis 2019;16:E46.

7. The American Heart Association diet and lifestyle recommendations. Available at: https://www.heart.org/en/healthy-living/healthy-eating/eat-smart/nutrition-basics/aha-diet-and-lifestyle-recommendations. Accessed April 29, 2021.

8. Hansen-Krone IJ, Enga KF, Njølstad I, et al. Heart healthy diet and risk of myocardial infarction and venous thromboembolism. Thromb Haemost 2017;108(09):554–60.

9. Yang Q, Zhang Z, Gregg EW, et al. Added sugar intake and cardiovascular diseases mortality among US adults. JAMA Intern Med 2014;174(4):516–24.

10. Mathur K, Agrawal RK, Nagpure S, et al. Effect of artificial sweeteners on insulin resistance among type-2 diabetes mellitus patients. J Family Med Prim Care 2020;9(1):69.

11. Wang Y-J, Yeh T-L, Shih M-C, et al. Dietary sodium intake and risk of cardiovascular disease: a systematic review and dose-response meta-analysis. Nutrients 2020;12(10). https://doi.org/10.3390/nu12102934.

12. Al-Shaar L, Satija A, Wang DD, et al. Red meat intake and risk of coronary heart disease among US men: prospective cohort study. BMJ 2020;371. https://doi.org/10.1136/bmj.m4141.

13. Ha V, Sievenpiper JL, de Souza RJ, et al. Effect of dietary pulse intake on established therapeutic lipid targets for cardiovascular risk reduction: a systematic review and meta-analysis of randomized controlled trials. CMAJ 2014;186(8):E252–62.

14. Polak R, Phillips EM, Campbell A. Legumes: health benefits and culinary approaches to increase intake. Clin Diabetes 2015;33(4):198.

15. Maphosa Y, Jideani VA. The role of legumes in human nutrition. Functional food - improve health through adequate food. Published online 2017. Available at: https://www.google.com/books/edition/Functional_Food/-vyPDwAAQBAJ?hl=en&gbpv=0.

16. Bazzano LA, He J, Ogden LG, et al. Legume consumption and risk of coronary heart disease in US men and women: NHANES I Epidemiologic Follow-up Study. Arch Intern Med 2001;161(21):2573–8.

17. Kelemen LE, Kushi LH, Jacobs DR, et al. Associations of dietary protein with disease and mortality in a prospective study of postmenopausal women. Am J Epidemiol 2005;161(3). https://doi.org/10.1093/aje/kwi038.

18. Kim SJ, de Souza RJ, Choo VL, et al. Effects of dietary pulse consumption on body weight: a systematic review and meta-analysis of randomized controlled trials. Am J Clin Nutr 2016;103(5). https://doi.org/10.3945/ajcn.115.124677.

19. Pawlak R, Parrott SJ, Raj S, et al. How prevalent is vitamin B(12) deficiency among vegetarians? Nutr Rev 2013;71(2):110–7.

20. Zurbau A, Au-Yeung F, Blanco Mejia S, et al. Relation of different fruit and vegetable sources with incident cardiovascular outcomes: a systematic review and meta-analysis of prospective cohort studies. J Am Heart Assoc 2020;9(19). https://doi.org/10.1161/JAHA.120.017728.

21. Miller V, Mente A, Dehghan M, et al. Fruit, vegetable, and legume intake, and cardiovascular disease and deaths in 18 countries (PURE): a prospective cohort study. Lancet 2017;390(10107):2037–49.

22. Temple NJ. Fat, sugar, whole grains and heart disease: 50 years of confusion. Nutrients 2018;10(1). https://doi.org/10.3390/nu10010039.

23. Li Y, Hruby A, Bernstein AM, et al. Saturated fats compared with unsaturated fats and sources of carbohydrates in relation to risk of coronary heart disease: a prospective cohort study. J Am Coll Cardiol 2015;66(14). https://doi.org/10.1016/j.jacc.2015.07.055.

24. Suggested servings from each food group. Available at: https://www.heart.org/en/healthy-living/healthy-eating/eat-smart/nutrition-basics/suggested-servings-from-each-food-group. Accessed April 5, 2021.

25. Sacks FM, Carey VJ, Anderson CAM, et al. Effects of high vs low glycemic index of dietary carbohydrate on cardiovascular disease risk factors and insulin sensitivity: the OmniCarb randomized clinical trial. JAMA 2014;312(23):2531–41.

26. Reynolds A, Mann J, Cummings J, et al. Carbohydrate quality and human health: a series of systematic reviews and meta-analyses. Lancet 2019;393(10170): 434–45.

27. Sacks FM, Lichtenstein AH, Wu JHY, et al. Dietary fats and cardiovascular disease: a presidential advisory from the American Heart Association. Circulation 2017;136(3). https://doi.org/10.1161/CIR.0000000000000510.

28. Mozaffarian D, Micha R, Wallace S. Effects on coronary heart disease of increasing polyunsaturated fat in place of saturated fat: a systematic review and meta-analysis of randomized controlled trials. PLoS Med 2010;7(3). https://doi.org/10.1371/journal.pmed.1000252.

29. Pallazola VA, Davis DM, Whelton SP, et al. A clinician's guide to healthy eating for cardiovascular disease prevention. Mayo Clin Proc Innov Qual Outcomes 2019; 3(3):251–67.

30. Naini AE, Keyvandarian N, Mortazavi M, et al. Effect of omega-3 fatty acids on blood pressure and serum lipids in continuous ambulatory peritoneal dialysis patients. Am J Pharmacogenomics 2015;4(3):135–41.

31. Burr ML, Fehily AM, Gilbert JF, et al. Effects of changes in fat, fish, and fibre intakes on death and myocardial reinfarction: diet and reinfarction trial (DART). Lancet 1989;2(8666):757–61.

32. Zong G, Li Y, Wanders AJ, et al. Intake of individual saturated fatty acids and risk of coronary heart disease in US men and women: two prospective longitudinal cohort studies. BMJ 2016;355. https://doi.org/10.1136/bmj.i5796.

33. Dehghan M, Mente A, Rangarajan S, et al. Association of dairy intake with cardiovascular disease and mortality in 21 countries from five continents (PURE): a prospective cohort study. Lancet 2018;392(10161). https://doi.org/10.1016/S0140-6736(18)31812-9.

34. Engel S, Tholstrup T. Butter increased total and LDL cholesterol compared with olive oil but resulted in higher HDL cholesterol compared with a habitual diet. Am J Clin Nutr 2015;102(2):309–15.

35. Martínez-González MA, Gea A, Ruiz-Canela M. The Mediterranean diet and cardiovascular health. Circ Res 2019;124(5):779–98.

36. Buil-Cosiales P, Toledo E, Salas-Salvadó J, et al. Association between dietary fibre intake and fruit, vegetable or whole-grain consumption and the risk of CVD: results from the PREvención con DIeta MEDiterránea (PREDIMED) trial. Br J Nutr 2016;116(3):534–46.

37. Hayes J, Benson G. What the latest evidence tells us about fat and cardiovascular health. Diabetes Spectr 2016;29(3):171–5.

38. Grosso G, Marventano S, Yang J, et al. A comprehensive meta-analysis on evidence of Mediterranean diet and cardiovascular disease: are individual components equal? Crit Rev Food Sci Nutr 2017;57(15):3218–32.

39. de Lorgeril Michel, Patricia Salen, Jean-Louis Martin, et al. Mediterranean diet, traditional risk factors, and the rate of cardiovascular complications after myocardial infarction. Circulation 1999;99(6):779–85.
40. Tognon G, Lissner L, Sæbye D, et al. The Mediterranean diet in relation to mortality and CVD: a Danish cohort study. Br J Nutr 2014;111(1):151–9.
41. Ornish D, Scherwitz LW, Billings JH, et al. Intensive lifestyle changes for reversal of coronary heart disease. JAMA 1998;280(23):2001–7.
42. Dansinger ML, Gleason JA, Griffith JL, et al. Comparison of the Atkins, Ornish, Weight Watchers, and Zone diets for weight loss and heart disease risk reduction: a randomized trial. JAMA 2005;293(1):43–53.
43. Li Z, Heber D. The Pritikin diet. JAMA 2020;323(11):1104.
44. Hartman AL, Vining EPG. Clinical aspects of the ketogenic diet. Epilepsia 2007; 48(1):31–42.
45. Weber DD, Aminzadeh-Gohari S, Tulipan J, et al. Ketogenic diet in the treatment of cancer - where do we stand? Mol Metab 2020;33:102–21.
46. Paoli A, Mancin L, Bianco A, et al. Ketogenic diet and microbiota: friends or enemies? Genes 2019;10(7). https://doi.org/10.3390/genes10070534.
47. Hall KD, Guo J, Courville AB, et al. Effect of a plant-based, low-fat diet versus an animal-based, ketogenic diet on ad libitum energy intake. Nat Med 2021;27(2): 344–53.
48. Lindeberg S, Jönsson T, Granfeldt Y, et al. A Palaeolithic diet improves glucose tolerance more than a Mediterranean-like diet in individuals with ischaemic heart disease. Diabetologia 2007;50(9):1795–807.
49. Osterdahl M, Kocturk T, Koochek A, et al. Effects of a short-term intervention with a paleolithic diet in healthy volunteers. Eur J Clin Nutr 2008;62(5):682–5.
50. Andrikopoulos S. The Paleo diet and diabetes. Med J Aust 2016;205(4):151–2.
51. Estruch R, Ros E, Salas-Salvadó J, et al. Primary prevention of cardiovascular disease with a Mediterranean diet supplemented with extra-virgin olive oil or nuts. N Engl J Med 2018;378(25):e34.
52. Sullivan S, Samuel S. Effect of short-term Pritikin diet therapy on the metabolic syndrome. J Cardiometab Syndr 2006;1(5):308–12.
53. Barnard R, Guzy P, Rosenberg J, et al. Effects of an intensive exercise and nutrition program on patients with coronary artery disease: five-year follow-up. Eur J Cardiovasc Prev Rehabil 1983;3(3):183–94.
54. Masood W, Annamaraju P, Uppaluri KR. Ketogenic diet. In: StatPearls. Treasure Island, Florida: StatPearls Publishing; 2020.
55. Rydhög B, Granfeldt Y, Frassetto L, et al. Assessing compliance with Paleolithic diet by calculating Paleolithic diet fraction as the fraction of intake from Paleolithic food groups. Clin Nutr Exp 2019;25:29–35.
56. Clark JE. Diet, exercise or diet with exercise: comparing the effectiveness of treatment options for weight-loss and changes in fitness for adults (18-65 years old) who are overfat, or obese; systematic review and meta-analysis. J Diabetes Metab Disord 2015;14:31.
57. Foster-Schubert KE, Alfano CM, Duggan CR, et al. Effect of diet and exercise, alone or combined, on weight and body composition in overweight-to-obese postmenopausal women. Obesity 2012;20(8):1628–38.
58. Wilkinson MJ, Manoogian ENC, Zadourian A, et al. Ten-hour time-restricted eating reduces weight, blood pressure, and atherogenic lipids in patients with metabolic syndrome. Cell Metab 2020;31(1):92–104.e5.
59. O'Connor SG, Boyd P, Bailey CP, et al. Perspective: time-restricted eating compared with caloric restriction: potential facilitators and barriers of long-term

weight loss maintenance. Adv Nutr 2021. https://doi.org/10.1093/advances/nmaa168.

60. Moro T, Tinsley G, Bianco A, et al. Effects of eight weeks of time-restricted feeding (16/8) on basal metabolism, maximal strength, body composition, inflammation, and cardiovascular risk factors in resistance-trained males. J Transl Med 2016;14(1). https://doi.org/10.1186/s12967-016-1044-0.

61. Tripp-Reimer T, Choi E, Kelley LS, et al. Cultural barriers to care: inverting the problem. Diabetes Spectr 2001;14(1):13–22.

62. Darmon N, Drewnowski A. Contribution of food prices and diet cost to socioeconomic disparities in diet quality and health: a systematic review and analysis. Nutr Rev 2015;73(10):643–60.

63. Ceasar JN, Claudel SE, Andrews MR, et al. Community engagement in the development of an mhealth-enabled physical activity and cardiovascular health intervention (Step It Up): Pilot Focus Group Study. JMIR Form Res 2019;3(1):e10944.

64. Colby S, Ortman JM, Others. Projections of the size and composition of the US population: 2014 to 2060. 2015. Available at: https://mronline.org/wp-content/uploads/2019/08/p25-1143.pdf. Accessed March 3, 2021.

65. Chesla CA, Kwan CML, Chun KM, et al. Gender differences in factors related to diabetes management in Chinese American immigrants. West J Nurs Res 2014;36(9):1074–90.

66. Juraschek SP, Miller ER 3rd, Weaver CM, et al. Effects of sodium reduction and the DASH diet in relation to baseline blood pressure. J Am Coll Cardiol 2017;70(23):2841–8.

67. Appel LJ, Moore TJ, Obarzanek E, et al. A clinical trial of the effects of dietary patterns on blood pressure. DASH Collaborative Research Group. N Engl J Med 1997;336(16):1117–24.

68. Hodson L, Harnden KE, Roberts R, et al. Does the DASH diet lower blood pressure by altering peripheral vascular function? J Hum Hypertens 2010;24(5):312–9.

69. Rice Bradley BH. Dietary fat and risk for type 2 diabetes: a review of recent research. Curr Nutr Rep 2018;7(4):214.

The Role of Physical Activity and Exercise in Preventive Cardiology

Paul D. Thompson, MD[a,b,*]

KEYWORDS

- Physical activity • Exercise • Exercise training • Coronary disease
- Atherosclerotic risk factors • Angina • Claudication

KEY POINTS

- Increased physical activity is associated with an approximately 50% reduction in cardiac events between the least and most active individuals.
- Exercise rarely cures a markedly abnormal cardiac risk factor but is excellent adjunctive treatment of dyslipidemia, hypertension, glucose intolerance, and increased body weight.
- Exercise-based cardiac rehabilitation should be recommended to essentially all patients after a myocardial infarction, valve or bypass surgery, or the diagnosis of heart failure.
- Walking is an effective treatment of claudication in patients without critical limb ischemia.

INTRODUCTION

My preventive clinical cardiology career started in 1978 after training in cardiology/preventive cardiology at the Stanford Heart Disease Prevention Program. I am not sure if other preventive cardiology training programs existed at that time, but I was attracted to the Stanford program because the faculty included Peter Wood, PhD and William Haskell, PhD. Dr Wood was the first to report that endurance athletes had markedly higher high-density lipoprotein (HDL) cholesterol levels[1]; Dr Haskell was a premier exercise physiologist. They were joined during my second year by Ralph Paffenbarger, MD, DrPH, principal investigator of the San Francisco Longshoreman[2] and subsequent Harvard Alumni[3] studies, both showing that more physically active individuals had fewer cardiovascular events. It was a different time. The drug treatment of hyperlipidemia consisted of clofibrate, bile acid sequestrants, and niacin. The drug treatment of diabetes consisted of insulin and sulfonylureas. I had never heard of coronary angioplasty until Andreas Gruentzig lectured at Stanford in

[a] Emeritus, Hartford Hospital, 80 Seymour Street Hartford, Hartford, CT 06070, USA;
[b] University of Connecticut
* Hartford Hospital, 80 Seymour Street Hartford, Hartford, CT 06070.
E-mail address: Paul.thompson@hhchealth.org

Med Clin N Am 106 (2022) 249–258
https://doi.org/10.1016/j.mcna.2021.11.002
0025-7125/22/© 2022 Elsevier Inc. All rights reserved.

1977 during my fellowship. I was terribly skeptical of the procedure, but one of my co-fellows, John Simpson, MD, was enthralled with the concept and visited Gruentzig in Switzerland. John returned convinced that he could invent a better catheter and with co-fellow Ned Roberts, MD launched an incredibly successful business career by inventing the Simpson/Roberts angioplasty catheter. In contrast to such inventions, exercise and physical activity (PA) have been advocated by expert clinicians since antiquity. Herodicus (480–? BC) was a Greek physician and martial arts teacher who integrated exercise and medicine.[4] Knowledge of exercise medicine has also advanced. There are more and better designed epidemiologic studies supporting the value of PA, and there is a better understanding of the basic science mechanisms by which exercise reduces atherosclerotic vascular disease (ASCVD) risk, but PA remains underutilized as a therapeutic modality. I last reviewed the role of exercise in cardiology in 2001.[5] The present article updates the previous report and reviews the value of exercise for preventing and treating ASCVD disease with an emphasis on what clinicians should know and do about exercise and PA.

PHYSICAL ACTIVITY, EXERCISE, AND CARDIORESPIRATORY FITNESS

Physical activity (PA) refers to any voluntary, bodily movement that burns calories. *Exercise* is PA "with a purpose" including to increase muscular strength, endurance, physical performance, or health. *Cardiorespiratory fitness* (CRF) is a measurement of the exercise performance capacity of the cardiovascular system. CRF is determined using exercises requiring large muscle groups such as treadmill walking or running, stationary cycling, or the time to walk or run a fixed distance. CRF is an indirect measurement of maximal oxygen uptake (VO_{2max}) or the maximal ability to consume oxygen during a specific exercise task. VO_{2max} is the product of maximal cardiac output (heart rate [HR] x stroke volume [SV]) and the maximal arterial-venous oxygen difference (A-VO2 Δ).[6] Because HR is largely age determined and the A-VO2 Δ varies relatively little among individuals, CRF is an indirect measurement of maximum SV. CRF increases with habitual PA and with exercise training, so it is often used as a measure of PA; this is an attractive approach because CRF is less variable than measurements of PA by self-report, but CRF is not a direct measure of PA. Other factors such as genetics and innate exercise capacity also affect CRF. I refer to this innate exercise capacity as the "hardiness factor" or the fact that some individuals are innately hardier and have increased CRF. And remember that increased CRF indicates an increased SV. CRF is one of the best predictors of reduced ASCVD risk and increased survival; this is attributed to PA in many studies, but it is important to acknowledge that this enhanced prognosis may be due to the hardiness factor and the larger stroke volume. Similar to the Timex watch commercial from the 1970s, subjects with increased CRF have a larger SV and a heart that can "take a licking and keep on ticking."

PHYSICAL ACTIVITY AND DECREASED ATHEROSCLEROTIC VASCULAR DISEASE RISK

PA is *associated* with decreased ACVD risk but has never been subjected to testing in healthy people to the most stringent form of medical evidence, the randomized, controlled clinical trial (RCCT). I was part of a group that performed what I think is the first comprehensive review of epidemiologic studies examining the relationship between PA and coronary artery disease (CAD).[7] We concluded that PA was inversely and causally related to a reduction in CAD and that CAD was approximately 50% lower in the highest versus the lowest physical activity groups. That study was initiated by Ken Powell, MD, a career-long, physical activity researcher at the Centers for Disease Control. I had published several early studies on sudden cardiac death (SCD) during vigorous exercise.[8,9] Dr Powell invited me to the Centers for Disease Control to debate Henry Solomon, MD the author of the book, *The Exercise Myth*.[10] Dr Solomon proposed that the danger of acute cardiac events during exercise outweighed its benefits, that people should exercise less vigorously, and that exercise did little to prevent CAD. This was a highly controversial topic when his book was published in 1984, given that interest in marathons and endurance exercise was exploding at the time. Indeed, there was a California pathologist, Dr Thomas Bassler, who had an incredible number of publications, composed almost entirely of letters to the editor, maintaining that running a marathon, a 42 km foot race, guaranteed protection against cardiac events, the so-called "Bassler Hypothesis."[11] My approach to the Solomon debate was to acknowledge that cardiac events did occur during exercise, since I had written about them,[8,9] but to emphasize that the benefits of physical activity outweighed the risk.

At that time there had never been, and likely there never will be, an RCCT comparing physical activity and sedentary behavior in previously healthy adults. Such a trial would require large numbers of subjects and would need to follow those subjects for a prolonged time. The number of subjects would need to be "huge," because the cardiac event rate in healthy subjects over a reasonable study duration would be low and also because there would be cross-overs from the PA group to the sedentary group and vice versa. At that time there had also never been, nor will there likely be, an RCCT of smoking versus nonsmoking, but Dr Luther L. Terry had already issued the first Surgeon General's report on smoking and health in 1964. Dr Terry determined that smoking caused adverse health outcomes by examining the relationship between smoking and health and epidemiologic characteristics. These included the strength of the relationship, its consistency study to study, whether it was appropriately sequenced meaning that smoking proceeded the disease and not the reverse, if there was a biological gradient in which more packs-per-day produced more disease, whether the relationship was biologically probable, and whether the relationship was coherent with all the facts.[12] These 5 criteria have since been criticized,[12] but I used them and a similar approach to the evidence in my debate with Dr Solomon. Dr Powell liked this approach and enlisted me and 2 of his colleagues to use epidemiologic data to conclude that PA reduces CAD.[7]

There have been multiple studies using more sophisticated techniques including meta-analysis since our publication.[13] These studies confirm that the risk of CAD is approximately 50% lower between the most and least active subjects. These studies also show that the greatest decrease in CVD is associated with increasing from the lowest to the next lowest PA cohort; this suggests that reductions in CAD events require only modest increases in physical activity. The lowest rate of CAD events is seen in the most active subjects, but the biggest decrease in CAD events occurs with only modest increases in PA[13]; this is partly because large portions of the population engage in no physical activity so that the population benefit is greatest with small increases in PA. These studies also show that CRF is a better predictor of CAD outcomes than PA, likely because CRF can be measured more accurately than the self-reported PA assessed in most trials but also because CRF measures the "hardiness factor" mentioned earlier.

HOW DOES PHYSICAL ACTIVITY REDUCE CORONARY ARTERY DISEASE EVENTS?

Exercise likely reduces CAD risk by multiple mechanisms. An analysis of subjects in the Women's Health Study demonstrated that compared with women self-reporting less than 200 kcal/wk of PA, the risk of CVD decreased 27%, 32%, and 41% as PA increased to 200 to 599, 600 to 1499, and greater than or equal to 1500 kcal/wk.[14]

Known risk factors (listed later) explained 59% of the CVD reduction. Inflammatory/hemostatic factors contributed the most, 32.6%, to the reduction, whereas blood pressure (−27.1%), total cholesterol (C), low-density lipoprotein cholesterol (LDL-C), HDL-C (−19.1%), lipoprotein (a) and apolipoproteins A-1 and B-100 (−15.5%), body mass index (−10.1%), and hemoglobin a1c/diabetes (−8.9%) contributed less. Why these risk factors add up to greater than 100% is unclear.

Many other exercise effects likely contribute. Exercise training lowers HR and increases parasympathetic or vagal tone. Every 10 beat per minute decrease in HR is associated with a 7% decrease in CHD and an 18% decrease in SCD.[15] Parasympathetic tone itself reduces cardiovascular risk. Exercise training in dogs increases HR variability, a marker of parasympathetic tone, and reduces the incidence of ischemia-induced ventricular fibrillation.[16] Exercise training increases coronary artery vasodilatory capacity and may increase coronary artery diameter. Runners who completed the Western States 100 miles run did not have larger coronary artery cross-sectional area at rest but did have markedly larger cross-sectional areas of their left anterior descending and circumflex coronary arteries after nitroglycerin administration.[17] Acetylcholine (ACH) produces vasoconstriction in atherosclerotic coronary arteries. Only 4 weeks of exercise training reduces this ACH vasoconstriction in patients with CAD.[18] The autopsy of Clarence DeMar, winner of 7 Boston Marathons, as reported by Currens and Paul Dudley White, the famous Boston cardiologist, showed extensive coronary atherosclerosis but large residual coronary lumens because of the coronaries' overall diameters.[19]

EXERCISE EFFECTS ON ATHEROSCLEROTIC VASCULAR DISEASE RISK FACTORS

Exercise affects multiple ASCVD risk factors, but exercise alone rarely cures clinically abnormal risk factors so should generally be viewed as adjunctive therapy. Exercise helps to control body weight and helps to prevent weight gain after weight loss but seems most useful for weight loss when combined with dietary caloric restriction.[20] Caloric expenditure during locomotive exercise is determined by the distance traveled and the body weight moved. The speed of locomotion matters because humans become less energy efficient with increased locomotive speed, but speed is less important than distance traveled and the grade of any elevation. Overweight individuals risk orthopedic injury with activities such as running. We recommend brisk walking to patients, rather than other exercises such as cycling or swimming, because the increased body weight of heavy individuals requires more caloric expenditure over the same distance than for a lighter person. I tell patients they can use their weight to "make lemonade out of their lemon."

Exercise can improve serum lipids. HDL cholesterol levels are 50% higher in endurance athletes, whereas triglycerides (TG) and LDL-C are approximately 50% and 10% lower, respectively.[21] Lipoprotein lipase activity (LPLA)[22] and intravenous fat clearance[23] are also higher in endurance athletes. Free fatty acids are a key energy source during endurance exercise. Using several marathons in Newport, RI as the laboratory, we demonstrated that exercise acutely reduces TGs and increases HDL-C[24,25] by increasing LPLA[25] and the clearance of intravenously administered fat.[25]

We postulated that decreased intramuscular fat from endurance exercise increases LPLA, which removes TGs from very low-density lipoproteins (VLDL).[21] The excess cholesterol on the VLDL surface that remains after TG removal is transferred to HDL by core lipid transport protein where it is esterified to increase HDL-C.[21] LDL-C is only slightly lower in endurance athletes possibly due to the expanded plasma volume that accompanies exercise training. Distance runners running 10 miles daily increased their LDL-C 10% within 2 days of exercise cessation[26] and decreased their plasma volume 5%,[27] suggesting that the expended plasma volume from training dilutes LDL-C. However, the newly available angiopoietin-like-3 (ANGPL3) monoclonal antibody, evinacumab, reduces LDL-C even in individuals lacking LDL receptors.[28] ANGPL3 inhibits LPLA, so increased LPLA from ANGPL3 inhibition suggests that the increased LPLA with acute exercise and exercise training may also contribute to lower LDL-C levels in very active subjects.

There is controversy about the role of HDL-C as a CVD risk factor because 2 trials of niacin therapy, which increases HDL-C, failed to demonstrate benefit, but in both instances, niacin was added to statin therapy. LDL-C levels at baseline in the AIM-HIGH[29] and the HPS-THRIVE[30] trials averaged only 72 and 63 mg/dL, making it difficult for niacin to demonstrate an effect. Other studies before statins were available, including the Coronary Drug Project using niacin[31] and the VA HDL Intervention Trial using gemfibrozil[32] did show reductions in CVD events and support the concept that HDL modification is important. Nevertheless, HDL-C remains the most predictive CAD lipid risk factor in many epidemiologic studies, so its increase with exercise is probably valuable.

I have focused on the effect of exercise on blood lipid because this was the focus of our National Institutes of Health–supported research for 11 years, but exercise also reduces systolic blood pressure[33] and improves insulin sensitivity[34] as well as many other risk factors.

Many of exercise's effects on risk factors are acute effects of recent exercise. TGs decrease within 24 hours of an exercise session.[35] Exercise acutely reduces systolic, and in some studies diastolic, blood pressure[36] likely from vasodilatation, and this reduction persists for up to 9 hours after exercise.[36] The average reduction in systolic blood pressure (SBP) and diastolic blood pressure (DBP) in subjects with prehypertension can be approximately 6 and 4 mm Hg, respectively, compared with the subjects' control session,[36] suggesting that the acute exercise effect is at least as powerful as some antihypertensive medicines.

Indeed, we have speculated that some of the risk factor effects attributed to exercise training are a cumulative effect of recent exercise. Exercise training increases fitness, which allows more exertion per session, which produces a larger acute effect when measured in fit subjects. At any rate, the observation that exercise produces an acute exercise effect argues for daily or at least frequent exercise to achieve the most beneficial effect on risk factors.

Despite the beneficial effect of exercise on CVD risk factors, it is important to recognize that exercise alone rarely normalized significantly abnormal risk factors. Patients need to know this because many delay effective drugs for long periods and are discouraged when their exercise efforts are insufficient.

EXERCISE-BASED CARDIAC REHABILITATION

Medicare approves exercise-based cardiac rehabilitation for patients after acute myocardial infarction, coronary revascularization, and valve surgery and for patients with angina pectoris and heart failure. The data are most robust for patients with CAD. A meta-analysis of 63 randomized control trials of exercise-based cardiac rehabilitation included 47 with mortality outcomes. These 47 studies followed 12, 455 patients for more than or equal to 6 months. Exercise-based rehab significantly reduced cardiac mortality in patients with CAD by 26% and hospital admissions by 18%.[37] Total mortality, MI, and revascularization were not significantly different between the rehab and control groups, although an earlier meta-analysis of 36 randomized trials including 6,111 patients post-MI found a 36% reduction in cardiac deaths, a 26%

reduction in total mortality, and a 47% reduction in reinfarction.[38] At least 2 observational studies of cardiac rehab including 846 and 3,975 patients after coronary artery bypass graft surgery (CABG) reported risk reductions of 46% and 40%.[38] Neither study was an RCCT, but both used propensity matching to try to adjust for selection bias. There are insufficient data to evaluate the effect of exercised-based rehab on patients after valve surgery, but the few available studies are supportive.

Exercise Training for Heart Failure

A meta-analysis of cardiac rehab in patients with heart failure and reduced ejection fraction (HFrEF) found that those randomized to rehab had a 45% reduction in mortality and a 28% reduction in death or hospital admission.[39] Medicare approval of rehab for HFrEF is largely based on HF-ACTION or the Heart Failure: A Controlled Trial Investigating Outcomes of Exercise Training, which randomized 2331 patients with HFrEF to exercise training or standard therapy.[40] All-cause mortality and hospitalization was reduced by 11% (P = .03) after adjustment for the prespecified baseline confounders of atrial fibrillation/flutter, psychological depression, ejection fraction, and exercise capacity. The secondary combined endpoint of cardiovascular mortality or HF hospitalizations was also reduced by 9% (P = .03) after adjustment for baseline variables. The investigators did nearly everything possible to keep the exercise-assigned patients actually exercising, including providing home exercise cycles or treadmills, but the increase in VO_{2max} in the training group was only 4%; this suggests that many of the exercise training participants did very little exercise training and that the benefits in patients with HFrEF could be significantly greater if patients would exercise.

Exercise Training for Angina Pectoris

Classic stable angina has essentially disappeared from modern cardiology because of β-blocker therapy, angioplasty, and CABG. Exercise-based therapy was an extremely useful therapy for stable angina and remains an underutilized adjunctive treatment for those patients who are not candidates for revascularization or who have symptoms despite medicines and revascularization. William Heberden, the English physician who first described angina, stated that he knew a patient who sawed wood for half an hour daily and was "nearly cured."[6] Medical historians think that Heberden was knowledgeable about the disease and the effects of exercise training because he was both physician and patient.

At least 2 factors contribute to the reduction in angina with exercise training.[6] HR is the primary determinant of myocardial oxygen demand. Exercise training reduces the HR response to any exercise workload so that after exercise training the patient can perform more exercise work before the onset of symptoms. Exercise training also improves abnormal endothelial function. Normal coronary arteries vasodilate with exercise, but atherosclerosis injures the endothelium so that the normal coronary vasodilatory response to exercise either does not occur or the arteries vasoconstrict. Reducing this exercise-induced vasoconstriction increases coronary blood flow and exercise capacity; this should not be interpreted as indicating that exercise is a replacement for modern medical therapy but that exercise training is valuable as adjunctive treatment of patients with angina who are not candidates for revascularization, refuse operative intervention, or have angina due to minor vessel disease.

Exercise Training for Claudication

Exercise training is an excellent treatment of claudication and has Medicare approval for this indication. Exercise training can produce remarkable increases in walking tolerance in patients who adhere to the program. An analysis of 25 RCCTs comparing walking exercise versus control found that the average increase in walking distance was 180 m.[41] Improvement in walking distance is greatest when walking is used as the exercise modality, patients walk to their maximal pain tolerance, and walking is pursued for greater than 6 months.[42] Another meta-analysis including stent revascularization found the greatest improvement with combined exercise and revascularization than with either therapy alone.[43] Patients need to know that the benefits of exercise on walking distance disappear with inactivity.

CLINICS CARE POINTS

The clinical implications of this review are as follows:

1. Clinicians should ask patients if they are physically active and for the specifics of the patient's activity program. Some have recommended that exercise be considered a vital sign for patient visits.[44] Many patients think that if the doctor does not ask it cannot be important.

2. Clinicians should know the 2018 Physical Activity Guidelines for Americans in order to advise patients to achieve at least the minimal recommended activity.[45] These guidelines recommend the following: move more/sit less, accumulate 150 to 300 min/wk of moderately vigorous exercise such as brisk walking or 75 to 150 min/wk of vigorous exercise such as jogging plus 2 resistance exercise sessions weekly to maintain muscle strength.

3. Exercise alone rarely normalizes a seriously abnormal cardiac risk factor, but exercise training is excellent adjunctive therapy for many cardiac risk factors including abnormal lipids, hypertension, excess body weight, and diabetes.

4. Clinician should be involved in advocating for physically active lifestyles in their community. Such advocating could be for walking paths, bicycle lanes, facility access, and other environmental engineering changes that enhance the population's ability to exercise. Jerry Morris, the British epidemiologist who led physical activity and outcomes studies of London bus drivers and conductors, called exercise "The best bargain in public health."[46] Clinicians should do what they can to make this bargain easily available to the public.

5. Clinicians should do their best to remove barriers from exercise participation; this includes not recommending exercise stress tests before starting a gradually progressive exercise program unless there are worrisome clinical symptoms. Exercise stress tests have long been known to predict angina and not SCD or acute MI (AMI). Positive exercise stress tests require ischemia from a significant coronary stenosis, whereas exercise-related SCD and AMI are usually produced by disruption of a previously nonobstructive lesion. Patients should be advised to promptly report new symptoms to the clinician but otherwise most patients can start exercise programs without undue risk.

6. All patients after AMI, valve or bypass surgery, or the diagnosis of HF should be referred to cardiac rehab. Utilization of cardiac rehabilitation is woefully low in the United States, and one of the biggest determinants as to whether or not a patient attends rehab is whether or not their clinician recommended it.

7. All patients with claudication in the absence of critical limb ischemia should be referred to a supervised exercise training program or advised to start a walking program on their own. Because maximal benefit is obtained when patients walk to maximal pain, I often recommend that patients buy a "cane chair" on the Internet so that they can walk to maximum pain, deploy the tripod cane chair, sit down to recover, and then walk again without having to find some other place to sit.

REFERENCES

1. Wood PD, Haskell W, Klein H, et al. The distribution of plasma lipoproteins in middle-aged male runners. Metabolism 1976;25:1249–57.

2. Paffenbarger RS, Laughlin ME, Gima AS, et al. Work activity of longshoremen as related to death from coronary heart disease and stroke. N Engl J Med 1970;282:1109–14.

3. Paffenbarger RS, Hyde RT, Wing AL, et al. Physical activity, all-cause mortality, and longevity of college alumni. N Engl J Med 1986;314:605–13.

4. Thompson PD. D. Bruce Dill Historical lecture. Historical concepts of the athlete's heart. Med Sci Sports Exerc 2004;36:363.

5. Thompson PD, Moyna N. The therapeutic role of exercise in contemporary cardiology Cardiovascular Reviews & Reports. Cardiovasc Rev Rep 2001;22:279–80, 22:279-280, 282-284, 2001. 282-284.

6. Thompson D. Exercise Prescription and Proscription for Patients With Coronary Artery Disease. Circulation 2005;112:2354–63.

7. Powell KE, Thompson PD, Caspersen CJ, et al. Physical activity and the incidence of coronary heart disease. Annu Rev Public Health 1987;8:253–87.

8. Thompson PD, Stern MP, Williams P, et al. Death during jogging or running. A study of 18 cases. JAMA 1979;242:1265–7.

9. Thompson PD, Funk EJ, Carleton RA, et al. Incidence of death during jogging in Rhode Island from 1975 through 1980. JAMA 1982;247:2535–8.

10. Solomon HA. The exercise Myth. 1984. Harcourt Brace Jovanovich; 1984.

11. Bassler TJ. Coronary-artery disease in marathon runners. N Engl J Med 1980;302:57–8.

12. Burch PR. The surgeon general's "epidemiologic criteria for causality." A critique. J Chronic Dis 1983;36:821–36.

13. Eijsvogels TM, Molossi S, Lee DC, et al. Exercise at the Extremes: The Amount of Exercise to Reduce Cardiovascular Events. J Am Coll Cardiol 2016;67:316–29.

14. Mora S, Cook N, Buring JE, et al. Physical activity and reduced risk of cardiovascular events: potential mediating mechanisms. Circulation 2007;116:2110–8.

15. Aune D, Sen A, o'Hartaigh B, et al. Resting heart rate and the risk of cardiovascular disease, total cancer, and all-cause mortality - A systematic review and dose-response meta-analysis of prospective studies. Nutr Metab Cardiovasc Dis 2017;27:504–17.

16. Hull SS, Vanoli E, Adamson PB, et al. Exercise training confers anticipatory protection from sudden death during acute myocardial ischemia. Circulation 1994;89:548–52.

17. Haskell WL, Sims C, Myll J, et al. Coronary artery size and dilating capacity in ultradistance runners. Circulation 1993;87:1076–82.

18. Hambrecht R, Wolf A, Gielen S, et al. Effect of exercise on coronary endothelial function in patients with coronary artery disease. N Engl J Med 2000;342:454–60.

19. CURRENS JH, WHITE PD. Half a century of running. Clinical, physiologic and autopsy findings in the case of Clarence DeMar ("Mr. Marathon"). N Engl J Med 1961;265:988–93.

20. Donnelly JE, Blair SN, Jakicic JM, et al. American College of Sports Medicine Position Stand. Appropriate physical activity intervention strategies for weight loss and prevention of weight regain for adults. Med Sci Sports Exerc 2009;41:459–71.

21. Thompson PD. What do muscles have to do with lipoproteins? Circulation 1990;81:1428–30.

22. Herbert PN, Bernier DN, Cullinane EM, et al. High-density lipoprotein metabolism in runners and sedentary men. JAMA 2021;252:1034–7.

23. Sady SP, Cullinane EM, Saritelli A, et al. Elevated high-density lipoprotein choles-terol in endurance athletes is related to enhanced plasma triglyceride clearance. Metabolism 1988;37:568–72.

24. Thompson PD, Cullinane E, Henderson LO, et al. Acute effects of prolonged ex-ercise on serum lipids. Metabolism 1980;29:662–5.

25. Sady SP, Thompson PD, Cullinane EM, et al. Prolonged exercise augments plasma triglyceride clearance. JAMA 1986;256:2552–5.

26. Thompson PD, Cullinane EM, Eshleman R, et al. The effects of caloric restriction or exercise cessation on the serum lipid and lipoprotein concentrations of endur-ance athletes. Metabolism 1984;33:943–50.

27. Cullinane EM, Sady SP, Vadeboncoeur L, et al. Cardiac size and VO2max do not decrease after short-term exercise cessation. Med Sci Sports Exerc 1986;18:420–4.

28. Raal FJ, Rosenson RS, Reeskamp LF, et al. Evinacumab for homozygous familial hypercholesterolemia. N Engl J Med 2020;383:711–20.

29. AIM-HIGH Investigators, Boden WE, Probstfield JL, et al. Niacin in patients with low HDL cholesterol levels receiving intensive statin therapy. N Engl J Med 2011;365:2255–67.

30. HPS2-THRIVE Collaborative Group, Landray MJ, Haynes R, et al. Effects of extended-release niacin with laropiprant in high-risk patients. N Engl J Med 2014;371:203–12.

31. Canner PL, Berge KG, Wenger NK, et al. Fifteen year mortality in Coronary Drug Project patients: long-term benefit with niacin. J Am Coll Cardiol 1986;8:1245–55.

32. Rubins HB, Robins SJ. Conclusions from the VA-HIT study. Am J Cardiol 2000;86:543–4.

33. Boutcher YN, Boutcher SH. Exercise intensity and hypertension: what's new? J Hum Hypertens 2017;31:157–64.

34. Goodyear LJ, Kahn BB. Exercise, glucose transport, and insulin sensitivity. Annu Rev Med 1998;49:235–61.

35. Cullinane E, Siconolfi S, Saritelli A, et al. Acute decrease in serum triglycerides with exercise: is there a threshold for an exercise effect? Metabolism 1982;31:844–7.

36. Ash GI, Taylor BA, Thompson PD, et al. The antihypertensive effects of aerobic versus isometric handgrip resistance exercise. J Hypertens 2017;35:291–9.

37. Anderson L, Oldridge N, Thompson DR, et al. Exercise-based cardiac rehabilita-tion for coronary heart disease: cochrane systematic review and meta-analysis. J Am Coll Cardiol 2016;67:1–12.

38. McMahon SR, Ades PA, Thompson PD. The role of cardiac rehabilitation in pa-tients with heart disease. Trends Cardiovasc Med 2017;27:420–5.

39. Piepoli MF, Davos C, Francis DP, et al, ExTraMATCH Collaborative. Exercise training meta-analysis of trials in patients with chronic heart failure (ExTra-MATCH). BMJ 2004;328:189.

40. O'Connor CM, Whellan DJ, Lee KL, et al. Efficacy and safety of exercise training in patients with chronic heart failure: HF-ACTION randomized controlled trial. JAMA 2009;301:1439–50.

41. McDermott MM. Exercise training for intermittent claudication. J Vasc Surg 2017;66:1612–20.

42. Gardner AW, Poehlman ET. Exercise rehabilitation programs for the treatment of claudication pain. A meta-analysis. JAMA 1995;274:975–80.

43. Saratzis A, Paraskevopoulos I, Patel S, et al. Supervised exercise therapy and revascularization for intermittent claudication: network meta-analysis of randomized controlled trials. JACC Cardiovasc Interv 2019;12:1125–36.

44. Golightly YM, Allen KD, Ambrose KR, et al. Physical activity as a vital sign: a systematic review. Prev Chronic Dis 2017;14:E123.

45. Piercy KL, Troiano RP, Ballard RM, et al. The physical activity guidelines for Americans. JAMA 2018;320:2020–8.

46. Morris JN. Exercise in the prevention of coronary heart disease: today's best buy in public health. Med Sci Sports Exerc 1994;26:807–14.

Update in Hypertension

Christopher B. McFadden, MD

KEYWORDS

- Hypertension (HTN) • Blood pressure • White coat hypertension • ACC guidelines

KEY POINTS

- Blood Pressure (BP) reduction improves cardiovascular (CV) outcomes.
- BP measurement techniques have evolved over time.
- Close attention to BP measurement techniques is essential in the treatment of hypertension (HTN).
- HTN therapy should consider future CV event risk.

INTRODUCTION

Hypertension (HTN) is a common finding in adults in the Western world. Current estimates place the prevalence of HTN in the United States, when defined as a blood pressure (BP) of 130/80, as 45%.[1] The prevalence rate in non-Hispanic black patients was notably higher at 57%. Over the last 50 years, a series of intervention trials has demonstrated convincing cardiovascular (CV) benefits when BP was reduced using a variety of anti-HTN medications. In addition to a drop in target BP, there has been significant developments in the devices used to measure BP during this period. Importantly, we now recognize several key components when considering how to measure and treat elevations in BP. The first is the concept that office BP measurements do not predict CV risk as well as other measurements. CV risk reduction is the primary benefactor of anti-HTN treatment; considering this, it is now clear the best obtainable measure of BP should be used to initiate and monitor treatment success. The second development is the concept that different individuals have different future CV risk; HTN therapy should take this into account. Recent guidelines include an assessment of CV risk when deciding BP targets. For this review, we will specifically comment on BP reduction's impact on CV risk in the following important groups of patients: those with chronic kidney disease (CKD), elderly subjects, and those with diabetes mellitus (DM). In addition, we will provide an overview of different BP measurement techniques.

BLOOD PRESSURE MEASUREMENTS

Measurement accuracy of BP is a key component in the assessment and treatment of HTN. We now understand traditional office BP measurements misrepresent overall BP

Department of Medicine, Cooper Medical School of Rowan University, 401 Haddon Avenue, Room 280, Camden, NJ 08103, USA
E-mail address: mcfadden-christopher@cooperhealth.edu

Med Clin N Am 106 (2022) 259–267
https://doi.org/10.1016/j.mcna.2021.11.003
0025-7125/22/© 2021 Elsevier Inc. All rights reserved.

levels due to consistent measurement irregularities due to poor technique as well as the changes in BP that occur as individuals enter into health care settings. This effect is termed white coat effect or white coat HTN depending on the presence or absence of a diagnosis of HTN, respectively. Too often, patients are not given adequate time to rest, are not measured with an adequately sized cuff, are not positioned in seated environment with leg and back support, or are talking during measurements. All of these can elevate BP; a nonstandardized BP measurement such as this is called routine or casual. In comparison, BP measurements obtained in clinical studies use protocols that are not consistently practiced in routine clinical settings. Checklists emphasizing BP techniques can improve the accuracy of BP readings and should be implemented; home BP measurement accuracy improves with the use of checklists as well.[2]

As previously stated, alternative BP measurements are now recognized as superior to traditional, routine office BP measurements.[3] These are home BP measurements, automated office BP (AOBP) measurements, and ambulatory BP measurements as well as more rigorous (research quality) office BP measurements. **Table 1** summarizes the average differences these readings will yield compared with a current study standard, AOBP, in patients with HTN. From a practical viewpoint, one should use the most accurate BP measurement available and have a low threshold to obtain out-of-office BP measurements to support ongoing HTN treatment. Current guidelines support and, in fact, emphasize the use of home and ambulatory BP monitoring to verify BP readings obtained in the office.[2,4] An essential component of both home- and office-based BP readings is proper technique and device validation. Finally, techniques using oscillometric techniques measure mean arterial pressure and calculate systolic and diastolic pressures; they may be less accurate in the setting of atrial arrhythmias, although evidence suggests repeated measurements, *if done*, may minimize this difference.[5] Techniques using oscillometric BP measurements include AOBP devices, home BP using automated devices, ABP, and office BP using automated devices. Thus, one isolated BP reading without being repeated is almost an unactionable value.

Table 1
Difference in systolic blood pressure readings compared with automated office blood pressure in individuals with hypertension[6–8]

	Pros	Cons	Difference from AOBP	Notable Facts—Including Outcome Studies
Routine Office BP	Ease of use	White coat effect User error	+ 14.5 mm Hg	
Research Office BP	More accurate	Time commitment	+ 7 mm Hg	Extra training
Automated Office BP	Reduce WCH/WCE	New device reqd. Time commitment	Reference	Used in SPRINT and ACCORD
Home BP	Reduce WCH/WCE Patient empowerment	Technique may be different Access variable Machine validation necessary	+ 2.6 mm Hg	Commonly used
Ambulatory BP (awake)	ABP (24 h) best future CV prediction	Access limited	+ 0.3 mm Hg	Night time BP monitoring possible

OUTCOMES IN SPECIAL POPULATIONS: CHRONIC KIDNEY DISEASE

CKD is defined as an abnormality in kidney structure or function, as evidenced by an estimated glomerular filtration rate (eGFR) of less than 60 mL/min/m^2 or urine albumin/creatinine ratio of greater than 30 mg/g, with implications for health.[9] Within the population of patients with CKD, HTN is very common. A review of participants in a large cohort of patients with CKD with eGFRs between 20 and 70 mL/min showed a HTN prevalence rate of 85%.[10] Proposed mechanisms for the high incidence of HTN in the CKD population include enhanced sodium reabsorption by damaged kidneys, upregulated renin-angiotensin as well as sympathetic nervous system activity, and a reduction in vasodilator presence.[11–13] Stage 3a CKD without albuminuria, particularly in elderly subjects, is a group with unclear CV risks related to kidney disease. Conversely, albuminuria, at all levels of kidney disease, is associated with an increased CV risk even at levels less than the traditional threshold for microalbuminuria (30 mg/g of creatinine).[14]

The 2017 American Heart Association guidelines state the BP goal for subjects with CKD should be less than 130/80 mm Hg. This recommendation is the strongest recommendation possible (class 1) within these guidelines. This recommendation is largely derived from the SPRINT study.[15] Within SPRINT, 28% of enrollees had some form of CKD although DM at study initiation was an exclusion. The group randomized to the lower SBP target of less than 120 mm Hg, as determined by AOBP measurement, developed CV events over the subsequent 3 years at a rate of 1.65% per year compared with 2.19% per year in the control group, whose SBP target was less than 140 mm Hg. These results led to the early termination of the study. The more recent KDIGO 2021 HTN guidelines propose a general target for office systolic BP of 120 mm Hg, referencing that target in the Sprint trial.[16] Importantly these guidelines emphasize the importance of standardized, repeated measurements in the office to determine BP most accurately. Clearly, it is inappropriate to aim for BP targets when the measurement technique yields consistently higher numbers compared with the study from which the target BP is drawn, such as known to occur with typical or "casual" BP measurements. In that setting, individuals may have their BP pushed too low.

Achievement of BP goals within the CKD population, as well as most populations, requires a commitment to lifestyle modifications as well as a willingness to use multiple medications. Consistently, studies have shown dietary modification in the form of lower sodium intake can reduce BP.[17,18] Sodium intake reduction reduces BP and improves the effectiveness of BP mediations, in particular angiotensin-converting enzyme (ACE) inhibitors and angiotensin receptor blockers (ARB). A higher intake of potassium in the form of fruits and vegetables, as tolerated by serum potassium in this population, can also improve BP control. The following lifestyle interventions and the expected outcomes on SBP are described in the 2017 HTN guidelines.

Weight loss of 5 kg—5 mm Hg
Low sodium diet (1500–2000 mg/d)—5 mm Hg
High fruit/vegetable diet, such as DASH—11 mm Hg
Moderation in alcohol consumption—4 mm Hg
Regular aerobic exercise—5 mm Hg
High potassium diet (not in patients with CKD)—4 mm Hg

In addition to BP targets, certain medication classes may be more beneficial in terms of CV and/or kidney event outcomes. In particular, in the presence of albuminuria defined as greater than 300 mg/d or greater than 300 mg albumin/g creatinine, an ACE inhibitor or ARB should provide additional CV and/or kidney protection.

A summary of additional key HTN management principles in the CKD population includes the following:

1. Anti-HTN medication numbers often need to reach more than 3 medications to obtain BP control in patients with CKD; small trials suggest some benefit with 1+ medication given at bedtime
2. Secondary endpoints suggest ACE inhibitors may be beneficial at a lower proteinuria threshold in African-American patients[19]
3. Diuretic use is a key principle in managing HTN in patients with CKD
4. Thiazide medications have benefit less than eGFRs of 30 mL/min[20]
5. Torsemide is the loop diuretic with the longest duration of action; other loops will likely need twice a day dosing
6. An increase in creatinine is tolerable if volume overload/CHF symptoms improve[21]
7. Potassium binding agents may allow continued use of RAS active mediations with hyperkalemia. Outcome studies on this topic are lacking[22]
8. Proteinuria despite maximum dose ACE/ARB therapy can be treated with aldosterone antagonists or SGLT2 inhibitors

BLOOD PRESSURE IN THE ELDERLY

HTN is common in older individuals and typically manifests as systolic HTN.[23] The increase in SBP occurs from stiffening of large arterial walls related to changes in the intima, media, and extracellular matrix both independent of pathology (ie, age related) and associated with specific pathologic conditions.[24] The treatment of HTN in elderly subjects, defined as 65 years and older, is challenging. First, this represents a growing population with a high risk of imminent CV events but who also are at risk for effects of polypharmacy. Randomized trials have provided some guidance toward the treatment of HTN in elderly subjects. Although older, primarily nonrandomized studies suggested a variable CV risk with lower SBP in elderly subjects, particularly older than 70 years with CKD,[25,26] the results of several recent trials dispute this. Current data support a goal SBP of less than 150 mm Hg in ambulatory, noninstitutionalized subjects without other compelling indications for lower BP. The 150 mm Hg SBP target for subjects older than 60 years is also the goal proposed by the American Academy of Family Practice although those guidelines do recognize potential benefit of an SBP target less than 140 mm Hg in the presence of CV risk including stroke or transient ischemic attack.[27] Most elderly subjects are, of course, at high risk for a future CV event in the next 10 years and could be classified as the group to which the SPRINT trial outcomes are relevant (SBP target of 120 mm Hg group). A subgroup analysis of the SPRINT study limited to subjects older than 75 years suggested the lower SBP target was not harmful and, in fact, was beneficial in terms of a reduced CV with tolerable side effects.[28]

In addition to benefits in terms of reducing CV events, we now recognize better BP control in elderly subjects delays declines in cognitive function. In the SPRINT-MIND trial, dementia outcomes were not different in the intensive and nonintensive BP groups although cognitive deficits seemed to be less common in the intensive treatment group.[29] Secondary outcomes, however, did favor tighter control in terms of reduction in cognitive impairment and the combination of cognitive impairment and probable dementia. The DANTE study demonstrated no improvement in elderly subjects with HTN with mild cognitive impairment randomized to medication discontinuation.[30]

SPRINT-MIND and DANTE investigated the potential for BP reduction via medications to affect cognitive function in the elderly population, potentially negatively.

Elderly subjects are at risk for other side effects from medications including falls related to hypotension, acute kidney injury, and confusion. Because of efficacy and side effects, β-blockers should not be first-line therapy for HTN in elderly subjects without other compelling indication.[31] Consistently, studies have not shown increased risk of adverse events in elderly subjects related to lower BP in study settings.[32,33] How subjects perform in nonstudy settings and how they may feel in terms of tolerability of medications used, recognizing typical number needed to treat as 20 to 40 subjects over several years, is an area not well understood.

Elderly subjects show a high prevalence of white coat HTN.[34] In addition, as SBP is lowered toward goal, an untoward side effect may be the reduction in diastolic BP (DBP) to a level causing symptoms and signs of tissue underperfusion.[35] Outcomes studies about low DBP, following treatment of systolic HTN, are limited.

Finally, BP trials in elderly subjects consistently enroll ambulatory, noninstitutionalized subjects. As the results of these trials enter clinical practice, close attention will need to be paid to how an individual's functional status is doing and whether these same guidelines apply. The very frail population older than 80 years may be particularly unique, and regular consideration should be given to their ideal anti-HTN treatment.[36]

BLOOD PRESSURE AND DIABETES

Patients with DM develop CV events and microvascular damage at a rate far higher than the general population. Presumptively, then, interventions that lower CV events in the general population should have a greater impact on patients with DM. The Accord BP study disputed this presumption, as patients with DM did not have improved CV event rates when randomized to a goal SBP of less than 120 mm Hg as compared with less than 140 mm Hg as measured by an AOBP machine.[37] This study plays a large role in BP guidelines from the American Diabetes Association (ADA), which define the HTN threshold and general goal as less than 140/90 mm Hg unless high risk for CV disease. In that case, and presuming therapy is tolerated, the lower goal of less than 130/80 is proposed as potentially appropriate.[38] Because of the difference in BP threshold for HTN diagnosis, the prevalence rate of HTN within the DM population will be different. Even with the more conservative ADA definition, however, 66% of US patients with DM are hypertensive.[39]

Hyperglycemia and an increased insulin state in type 2 DM creates a state of volume expansion and, due to SNS alterations, upregulation of the renin-angiotensin system.[40] It is not surprising that diuretics and agents directed at the renin angiotensin system show the best impact on uncontrolled HTN in DM patients with DM. In patients with low levels of albuminuria, in the range 30 to 300 ug/mg creatinine, ACE or ARB therapy provides excellent BP control, particularly when combined with a diuretic. Their use in that setting is not superior to other classes of anti-HTN medications.[41] In addition to CV events, patients with DM suffer from a disproportionate share of kidney disease including progression to end-stage kidney failure. Yet, most patients with DM do not reach this endpoint even if albuminuria is present because of their even higher CV risk rate. As tempting as it is to consider patients with DM to benefit from the goals from the SPRINT trial, that trial did not enroll DM at baseline. Interpreting the competing outcomes of the SPRINT and ACCORD trials, particularly if patients are elderly, is an essential and challenging part of anti-HTN therapy. Ideally, providers should involve patients in the decisions about BP targets while including some discussion of risks and benefits of therapy, patient tolerability of medications, some descriptions of numbers needed to treat data, and providers' own recommendations. These are not simple conversations, and their conclusions may change over time as patients' health and medication tolerability change. Important considerations in the care of patients with DM include the following:

Outcome studies of BP control in patients with DM generally enroll patients with type 2 DM; high CV event rates in type 1 DM suggest similar BP benefits exist for this population

Lifestyle modifications should be a cornerstone of HTN therapy in subjects with DM and initiated when BP is greater than 120/80[38]

Hyperkalemia is a common finding in DM with HTN, particularly with ACE/ARB therapy and kidney disease; diuretics can improve this

The 2 new DM agents, SGLT2 and GLP-1 inhibitors, can reduce BP[42]

Thiazides may alter glucose metabolism modestly; studies do not suggest this has significant outcome differences[43]

SUMMARY

BP is a modifiable risk factor for future CV disease. The risk of events and the expected benefits from therapy are different for different individuals; thus, a "tailoring" of anti-HTN treatment uses an individual's risk for future CV events. In general, there has been a movement toward lower BP targets with a systolic target of 120 mm Hg existing for most individuals with CKD or higher risk for future CV disease in the next 10 years. Prescribers should understand the risk reduction attributable to reduction of BP for any given individual as they discuss this important therapeutic option with patients. A reassessment of targets and tolerability of therapy should regularly occur. Providers should regularly consider how to obtain the best BP measurement available. Often, this will be a combination of office readings, performed under standardized circumstances, and home BP measurements following education about proper techniques. The advantages of this approach are numerous including patient empowerment, identification of irregularities such as white coat HTN, and, most importantly, an expected improvement in the health of patients.

DISCLOSURE

The author has nothing to disclose.

REFERENCES

1. Statistics NCfH. National Health and Nutrition Examination Survey. Centers for Disease Control and Prevention. 2020. Available at: https://www.cdc.gov/nchs/data/factsheets/factsheet_nhanes.pdf. Accessed April 12, 2021, 2021.
2. Whelton PK, Carey RM, Aronow WS, et al. 2017 ACC/AHA/AAPA/ABC/ACPM/AGS/APhA/ASH/ASPC/NMA/PCNA Guideline for the Prevention, Detection, Evaluation, and Management of High Blood Pressure in Adults: A Report of the American College of Cardiology/American Heart Association Task Force on Clinical Practice Guidelines. J Am Coll Cardiol 2018;71(19):e127–248.
3. Myers MG. The great myth of office blood pressure measurement. J Hypertens 2012;30(10):1894–8.
4. Siu AL. Screening for high blood pressure in adults: U.S. Preventive Services Task Force recommendation statement. Ann Intern Med 2015;163(10):778–86.
5. Pagonas N, Schmidt S, Eysel J, et al. Impact of atrial fibrillation on the accuracy of oscillometric blood pressure monitoring. Hypertension 2013;62(3):579–84.

6. Myers MG, Godwin M, Dawes M, et al. Conventional versus automated measurement of blood pressure in primary care patients with systolic hypertension: randomised parallel design controlled trial. BMJ 2011;342:d286.
7. Lamarre-Cliché M, Cheong NN, Larochelle P. Comparative assessment of four blood pressure measurement methods in hypertensives. Can J Cardiol 2011; 27(4):455–60.
8. Roerecke M, Kaczorowski J, Myers MG. Comparing automated office blood pressure readings with other methods of blood pressure measurement for identifying patients with possible hypertension: a systematic review and meta-analysis. JAMA Intern Med 2019;179(3):351–62.
9. Stevens PE, Levin A. Evaluation and management of chronic kidney disease: synopsis of the kidney disease: improving global outcomes 2012 clinical practice guideline. Ann Intern Med 2013;158(11):825–30.
10. Muntner P, Anderson A, Charleston J, et al. Hypertension awareness, treatment, and control in adults with CKD: results from the Chronic Renal Insufficiency Cohort (CRIC) Study. Am J Kidney Dis 2010;55(3):441–51.
11. Passauer J, Pistrosch F, Büssemaker E, et al. Reduced agonist-induced endothelium-dependent vasodilation in uremia is attributable to an impairment of vascular nitric oxide. J Am Soc Nephrol 2005;16(4):959–65.
12. Neumann J, Ligtenberg G, Klein II, et al. Sympathetic hyperactivity in chronic kidney disease: pathogenesis, clinical relevance, and treatment. Kidney Int 2004;65(5):1568–76.
13. Ku E, Lee BJ, Wei J, et al. Hypertension in CKD: Core Curriculum 2019. Am J Kidney Dis 2019;74(1):120–31.
14. Matsushita K, van der Velde M, Astor BC, et al. Association of estimated glomerular filtration rate and albuminuria with all-cause and cardiovascular mortality in general population cohorts: a collaborative meta-analysis. Lancet 2010; 375(9731):2073–81.
15. Wright JT Jr, Williamson JD, Whelton PK, et al. A randomized trial of intensive versus standard blood-pressure control. N Engl J Med 2015;373(22):2103–16.
16. Cheung AK, Chang TI, Cushman WC, et al. Executive summary of the KDIGO 2021 clinical practice guideline for the management of blood pressure in chronic kidney disease. Kidney Int 2021;99(3):559–69.
17. Saran R, Padilla RL, Gillespie BW, et al. A randomized crossover trial of dietary sodium restriction in stage 3-4 CKD. Clin J Am Soc Nephrol 2017;12(3):399–407.
18. Garofalo C, Borrelli S, Provenzano M, et al. Dietary salt restriction in chronic kidney disease: a meta-analysis of randomized clinical trials. Nutrients 2018; 10(6):732.
19. Wright JT Jr, Bakris G, Greene T, et al. Effect of blood pressure lowering and antihypertensive drug class on progression of hypertensive kidney disease: results from the AASK trial. Jama 2002;288(19):2421–31.
20. Bovée DM, Visser WJ, Middel I, et al. A randomized trial of distal diuretics versus dietary sodium restriction for hypertension in chronic kidney disease. J Am Soc Nephrol 2020;31(3):650–62.
21. Metra M, Davison B, Bettari L, et al. Is worsening renal function an ominous prognostic sign in patients with acute heart failure? The role of congestion and its interaction with renal function. Circ Heart Fail 2012;5(1):54–62.
22. Agarwal R, Rossignol P, Romero A, et al. Patiromer versus placebo to enable spironolactone use in patients with resistant hypertension and chronic kidney disease (AMBER): a phase 2, randomised, double-blind, placebo-controlled trial. Lancet 2019;394(10208):1540–50.

23. Duprez DA. Systolic hypertension in the elderly: addressing an unmet need. Am J Med 2008;121(3):179–84.e3.

24. Lakatta EG. Arterial and cardiac aging: major shareholders in cardiovascular disease enterprises: Part III: cellular and molecular clues to heart and arterial aging. Circulation 2003;107(3):490–7.

25. Weiss JW, Peters D, Yang X, et al. Systolic BP and Mortality in Older Adults with CKD. Clin J Am Soc Nephrol 2015;10(9):1553–9.

26. Kovesdy CP, Alrifai A, Gosmanova EO, et al. Age and outcomes associated with BP in patients with incident CKD. Clin J Am Soc Nephrol 2016;11(5):821–31.

27. Hauk L. Pharmacologic Treatment of Hypertension: ACP and AAFP Release Recommendations for Adults 60 Years and Older. Am Fam Physician 2017;95(9):588–9.

28. Williamson JD, Supiano MA, Applegate WB, et al. Intensive vs standard blood pressure control and cardiovascular disease outcomes in adults aged ≥75 years: a randomized clinical trial. Jama 2016;315(24):2673–82.

29. Williamson JD, Pajewski NM, Auchus AP, et al. Effect of intensive vs standard blood pressure control on probable dementia: a randomized clinical trial. Jama 2019;321(6):553–61.

30. Moonen JE, Foster-Dingley JC, de Ruijter W, et al. Effect of discontinuation of antihypertensive treatment in elderly people on cognitive functioning–the DANTE Study Leiden: a randomized clinical trial. JAMA Intern Med 2015;175(10):1622–30.

31. James PA, Oparil S, Carter BL, et al. 2014 evidence-based guideline for the management of high blood pressure in adults: report from the panel members appointed to the Eighth Joint National Committee (JNC 8). Jama 2014;311(5):507–20.

32. Beckett NS, Peters R, Fletcher AE, et al. Treatment of hypertension in patients 80 years of age or older. N Engl J Med 2008;358(18):1887–98.

33. Staessen JA, Fagard R, Thijs L, et al. Randomised double-blind comparison of placebo and active treatment for older patients with isolated systolic hypertension. The Systolic Hypertension in Europe (Syst-Eur) Trial Investigators. Lancet 1997;350(9080):757–64.

34. Bulpitt CJ, Beckett N, Peters R, et al. Does white coat hypertension require treatment over age 80?: Results of the hypertension in the very elderly trial ambulatory blood pressure side project. Hypertension 2013;61(1):89–94.

35. Cruickshank JM. Coronary flow reserve and the J curve relation between diastolic blood pressure and myocardial infarction. Bmj 1988;297(6658):1227–30.

36. Benetos A, Bulpitt CJ, Petrovic M, et al. An expert opinion from the European Society of Hypertension-European Union Geriatric Medicine Society Working Group on the Management of Hypertension in Very Old, Frail Subjects. Hypertension 2016;67(5):820–5.

37. Cushman WC, Evans GW, Byington RP, et al. Effects of intensive blood-pressure control in type 2 diabetes mellitus. N Engl J Med 2010;362(17):1575–85.

38. 10. Cardiovascular Disease and Risk Management: Standards of Medical Care in Diabetes-2019. Diabetes Care 2019;42(Suppl 1):S103–23.

39. Shin D, Bohra C, Kongpakpaisarn K. Impact of the Discordance Between the American College of Cardiology/American Heart Association and American Diabetes Association recommendations on hypertension in patients with diabetes mellitus in the United States. Hypertension 2018;72(2):256–9.

40. Nosadini R, Sambataro M, Thomaseth K, et al. Role of hyperglycemia and insulin resistance in determining sodium retention in non-insulin-dependent diabetes. Kidney Int 1993;44(1):139–46.
41. de Boer IH, Bangalore S, Benetos A, et al. Diabetes and Hypertension: A Position Statement by the American Diabetes Association. Diabetes Care 2017;40(9): 1273–84.
42. Georgianos PI, Agarwal R. Ambulatory Blood Pressure Reduction With SGLT-2 Inhibitors: Dose-Response Meta-analysis and Comparative Evaluation With Low-Dose Hydrochlorothiazide. Diabetes Care 2019;42(4):693–700.
43. Barzilay JI, Davis BR, Pressel SL, et al. Long-term effects of incident diabetes mellitus on cardiovascular outcomes in people treated for hypertension: the ALL-HAT Diabetes Extension Study. Circ Cardiovasc Qual Outcomes 2012;5(2): 153–62.

Evaluation and Management of Secondary Hypertension

Harini Sarathy, MBBS, MHS[a,1], Liann Abu Salman, MD[b,1], Christopher Lee, MD[c], Jordana B. Cohen, MD, MSCE[d,e,*]

KEYWORDS

- Hypertension • Blood pressure • Secondary hypertension • Resistant hypertension
- Primary aldosteronism • Renal artery stenosis • Obstructive sleep apnea

KEY POINTS

- Secondary hypertension is common in patients with hypertension, particularly those diagnosed with hypertension at a young age or with resistant hypertension.
- Secondary hypertension merits evaluation to prevent target organ damage, but is often underrecognized.
- Appropriate evaluation of secondary hypertension depends largely on provider history taking to determine necessary testing.

INTRODUCTION

Hypertension is the leading cause of cardiovascular morbidity and premature death worldwide. The global prevalence of hypertension was estimated to be approximately 31% in 2010, affecting more than 1 billion persons worldwide.[1] Hypertension is typically described as essential, or primary, when there are no clearly discernible reasons for elevated blood pressure ($\geq$130/80 mm Hg).[2] Secondary hypertension, or hypertension that can be attributed to another underlying cause, is less common than primary hypertension, but is also underrecognized. Secondary hypertension often affects younger patients and those with resistant or refractory hypertension. Identifying the underlying

[a] Division of Nephrology and Hypertension, Zuckerberg San Francisco General Hospital, University of California San Francisco, 1001 Potrero Avenue, San Francisco, CA 94110, USA; [b] Renal-Electrolyte and Hypertension Division, Renal Division, Perelman School of Medicine, University of Pennsylvania, Hospital of the University of Pennsylvania, 3400 Spruce Street, 1 Founders, Philadelphia, PA 19104, USA; [c] Department of Medicine, Pennsylvania Hospital, University of Pennsylvania Health System, 800 Spruce Street, Philadelphia, PA 19104, USA; [d] Department of Biostatistics, Epidemiology, and Informatics, Perelman School of Medicine, University of Pennsylvania, 423 Guardian Drive, 831 Blockley, Philadelphia, PA 19104, USA; [e] Renal-Electrolyte and Hypertension Division, Perelman School of Medicine, University of Pennsylvania, Philadelphia, PA, USA
[1] Equal contributions.
* Corresponding author.
E-mail address: jco@pennmedicine.upenn.edu
Twitter: @hurryknee (H.S.); @LiannAbuSalman (L.A.S.); @LeetopherC (C.L.); @jordy_bc (J.B.C.)

Med Clin N Am 106 (2022) 269–283
https://doi.org/10.1016/j.mcna.2021.11.004
0025-7125/22/© 2021 Elsevier Inc. All rights reserved.
medical.theclinics.com

cause of secondary hypertension may lead to successful intervention with the potential to improve quality of life and reduce cardiovascular morbidity and mortality. Common secondary causes of hypertension include primary aldosteronism (PA), renovascular disease, chronic kidney disease, obstructive sleep apnea (OSA), and drug-induced or alcohol-induced hypertension. Rarer causes of secondary hypertension include catecholamine-secreting tumors (pheochromocytoma and paraganglioma), Cushing syndrome, hypothyroidism and hyperthyroidism, coarctation of aorta, and hyperparathyroidism. In this review, we focus on the identification and treatment of common causes of secondary hypertension and highlight the importance of obtaining a detailed history from the patient to facilitate appropriate diagnosis and treatment (**Table 1**).

DISCUSSION
Primary Aldosteronism

PA or Conn syndrome is the commonest form of secondary hypertension and is amenable to treatment if diagnosed appropriately.[3] Patients with PA have a significantly

Table 1
Presentation, evaluation, and management of common causes of secondary hypertension

Cause of Secondary Hypertension	Common Examples of Clinical Presentations	Evaluation	Management
PA	Resistant hypertension Hypokalemia and hypertension Adrenal mass Family history of early age of onset of hypertension	Plasma aldosterone concentration and renin activity or direct renin concentration Confirmatory testing by hypertension specialists Adrenal vein sampling	Unilateral disease: surgical resection Bilateral disease: mineralocorticoid receptor antagonist therapy
RVD	Resistant hypertension Abrupt onset hypertension Sudden worsening of blood pressure control Early age of onset of hypertension	Abdominal CT angiography (ideally); alternatively renal Doppler ultrasound examination (operator dependent) or magnetic resonance angiography	Medical optimization (preferred in atherosclerotic disease) Angioplasty with or without out stenting (preferred in FMD) Surgery (rare)
OSA	Resistant hypertension Witnessed apneic episodes while sleeping Daytime somnolence or fatigue	Polysomnography	Weight loss CPAP
Prescription or nonprescription substances	Resistant hypertension	Careful medication reconciliation Assessment of history of substance use	Discontinuation of offending agent and initiation of alternative therapy, if appropriate

increased risk of cardiovascular disease morbidity (including coronary heart disease, stroke, atrial fibrillation, left ventricular hypertrophy, heart failure, diabetes, and metabolic syndrome) and mortality compared with age- and sex-matched patients with essential or primary hypertension, and this risk is independent of degree of blood pressure control.[4] The elevated cardiovascular risk from PA is thought to be related to excessive stimulation of renal and extrarenal mineralocorticoid receptor activation, often causing fibrosis, endothelial dysfunction, and target organ damage. The early recognition of PA is crucial because treatment reliably lowers blood pressure, decreases the number of antihypertensive medications needed, and improves cardiac and renal function.

Although traditionally thought to be a rare form of hypertension that presents with severe hypertension with or without hypokalemia, recent evidence suggests that PA is present in up to 20% of patients with hypertension and is more common among those with greater severity of hypertension.[5–8] Nonetheless, screening for PA remains low and underused, even among patients with resistant hypertension.[9,10] PA is defined by autonomous and renin-independent, nonsuppressible aldosterone production, which results in excessive mineralocorticoid receptor activation and thus increased sodium reabsorption, hypertension, hypokalemia, and elevated risk of adverse cardiovascular outcomes. Autonomous aldosterone hypersecretion may occur from aldosterone-producing adenomas, idiopathic (often bilateral) adrenal hyperplasia (IAH), or abnormal aldosterone producing cell clusters present within morphologically normal adrenal glands.[5] Recent experimental and epidemiologic studies have demonstrated a continuous spectrum of renin-independent autonomous hyperaldosteronism, ranging from subtle to overtly autonomous aldosteronism, and that occurs in all stages of hypertension and even in normotensive individuals.[6,11] Consensus is still emerging whether all patients with hypertension should be screened for PA, regardless of the severity of the hypertension.

Screening for PA in primary care is easy, inexpensive, and noninvasive. Furthermore, screening for PA can potentially identify patients with treatable forms of hypertension and modify cardiovascular risk. Current guidelines recommend screening for PA in patients with severe hypertension and/or hypertension with hypokalemia (spontaneous or diuretic induced), particularly in those with resistant hypertension (defined as a blood pressure of >130/80 mm Hg despite being on 3 optimally dosed antihypertensive agents, of which one is a diuretic, or a blood pressure of <130/80 mm Hg with 4 antihypertensive agents), or associated with a family history of early-onset hypertension, stroke under the age of 40 years, a first-degree relative with PA, atrial fibrillation, sleep apnea, or adrenal incidentaloma.[2,5] Individuals who fall into these categories should have an aldosterone-to-renin ratio (ARR) measured, based on plasma aldosterone concentration and plasma renin activity or direct renin concentration. Guidelines recommend drawing the blood tests for aldosterone and renin levels about 2 hours after waking up in the morning and with the patient in the seated position. Because hypokalemia suppresses aldosterone production, potassium levels should be corrected to normal before screening. Ideally, patients should have unrestricted salt intake before testing to ensure volume expansion, and mineralocorticoid receptor antagonists (such as spironolactone) should be withdrawn for at least 4 weeks before testing. It is not essential for patients to remain off antihypertensive medications during testing, and it is often not safe to withhold antihypertensive medications in patients with moderate or severe hypertension.[2,5] Some recommendations suggest temporarily replacing antihypertensive agents with verapamil, hydralazine, or α-adrenergic blockers such as prazosin or doxazosin for the 4 weeks before testing, because these medications have minimal effects on plasma aldosterone or renin levels.[5] When it is not reasonably safe or feasible to discontinue diuretics, renin–angiotensin–aldosterone system inhibitors, or even mineralocorticoid receptor antagonists in patients with severe hypertension, testing is interpretable as long as renin levels are suppressed (which indicates volume expansion and therefore inhibition of endogenous feedback-driven aldosterone secretion).

ARR is a sensitive measure, but is not reliable by itself; it should be interpreted in the context of suppressed renin and elevated aldosterone levels. Patients with elevated ARR (>20) along with elevated plasma aldosterone levels (>10 ng/dL) and suppressed renin levels (plasma renin activity <1 ng/mL/h or direct renin concentration <10 pg/mL) are considered to have positive screening for biologically overt PA and then should undergo confirmatory testing for definitive diagnosis.[3,5] However, patients with spontaneous hypokalemia, suppressed renin, and a plasma aldosterone concentration of greater than 20 ng/dL are considered to have unequivocal PA from screening alone and can proceed directly to subtype classification (ie, to determine aldosterone-producing adenomas or unilateral IAH vs bilateral IAH).[5] Familial hyperaldosteronism (types I–IV) is a group of inherited PA disorders in patients with a significant family history of early onset hypertension and is associated with suppressed renin and elevated aldosterone levels, but a less elevated ARR compared with that seen with aldosterone-producing adenomas. Familial hyperaldosteronism can be identified with genetic testing.

Patients with positive screening should be referred to PA hypertension specialty care (depending on the practice, this can be endocrinology, nephrology, or cardiology) to undergo confirmatory testing before subtype classification.[5] Although there is no gold standard for confirmatory testing, 4 testing procedures are currently in common use across the world and are considered equivalent: (1) oral sodium loading, (2) saline infusion, (3) a fludrocortisone suppression test, which is more difficult to perform safely than the other options, and (4) a captopril challenge test, which is prone to equivocal results.[5] Most centers in the United States use oral sodium loading (>5 g/d for 3 days or a 2-L infusion of normal saline over 4 hours in a seated position) to induce volume expansion, which would normally suppress aldosterone production, but does not do so in patients with autonomous aldosterone production. Adequate salt loading with the oral test is verified by 24-hour urine collection on the third day of salt loading: urine sodium levels should be greater than 200 mmol/24 hours. A 24-hour urine aldosterone level of greater than 12 μg/24 hours after 3 days of oral salt loading or a serum aldosterone level of greater than 6 ng/dL after saline infusion confirms autonomous aldosterone production.

Subtype classification relies in noninvasive imaging with an adrenal computed tomography (CT) scan along with invasive adrenal vein sampling performed by an experienced interventional radiologist.[5] The initial adrenal CT scan can identify normal adrenal glands versus unilateral or bilateral macroadenoma (>1 cm) or microadenomas (≤1 cm), which present as hypodense nodules (<10 Hounsfield units, reflecting tissue that contains more lipid than water). It also excludes large masses (>4 cm) that would be suspicious for adrenocortical carcinoma. A CT scan is preferred over an MRI because it is less expensive and has better resolution. An adrenal CT scan also anatomically delineates the mass and adrenal venous anatomy that is crucial for adrenal vein sampling. IAH may seem to be normal on a CT scan or show nodular changes, and thus a CT scan alone is insufficient to delineate unilateral from bilateral disease. Adrenal vein sampling with lateralization of excessive aldosterone secretion is necessary to make that distinction so that treatment decisions can be made appropriately. Cosyntropin is often injected and cortisol and aldosterone levels are measure from each adrenal vein and compared with peripheral venous sampling. Adrenal vein sampling is a technically challenging procedure that requires an experienced operator, but is relatively safe.[12]

Depending on the PA subtype, unilateral laparoscopic adrenalectomy or mineralocorticoid receptor antagonist therapy can successfully treat and reverse the hypertension, hypokalemia, and excess cardiovascular risk imposed by autonomous aldosterone secretion.[2,3,5] Surgery is more effective than medications in patients with unilateral hypersecreting adrenal adenoma or unilateral IAH and is generally recommended unless the patient is unwilling or is not a surgical candidate. Patients with bilateral adrenal disease should be treated medically with a mineralocorticoid receptor antagonist both for blood pressure control and to protect against target organ damage from the effects of aldosterone that are independent of blood pressure control. Spironolactone remains the preferred initial agent, and should be started at low doses 12.5 to 25.0 mg/d and increased in 25-mg increments every 4 to 8 days to a maximum of 100 mg/d (although doses of ≤400 mg/d have been used).[3,5] The side effects of spironolactone are dose dependent and mainly in the form of gynecomastia and sexual dysfunction in men and menstrual irregularities and breast engorgement in women. Eplerenone, which is costlier and requires twice daily dosing, can be alternatives to spironolactone when side effects occur. Patients should be monitored for hyperkalemia, especially in those with impaired kidney function.

Renovascular Disease

Renovascular disease (RVD), often referred to as renal artery stenosis, is an important and potentially correctable cause of secondary hypertension that occurs in about 5% of individuals with a diagnosis of hypertension, with a higher prevalence among the elderly.[13,14] RVD results from decreased arterial blood flow to one or both kidneys leading to the overactivation of the renin–angiotensin–aldosterone system. In most cases, RVD is either caused by atherosclerosis (90%) or fibromuscular dysplasia (FMD) (9%) of the renal arteries.[15] Atherosclerotic RVD is commonly seen in patients age 50 or older, whereas FMD is more commonly seen in females less than 50 years of age.[16] Less common causes of RVD, not specifically addressed in this review, include renal artery aneurysm, systemic vasculitis, arteriovenous fistula, Page kidney (eg, owing to trauma to the kidney), renin-secreting tumors, aortic coarctation, and extrinsic compression of the renal artery.[17]

Risk factors for atherosclerotic RVD include an elevated low-density lipoprotein level, low high-density lipoprotein level, diabetes mellitus, hypertension, tobacco use, and the metabolic syndrome.[18] Approximately 80% to 90% of patients with FMD are female.[19,20] The development of FMD is likely related to a combination of genetic and environmental factors.[21] Environmental modifiers include female hormones, lifetime mechanical stress, and tobacco use. The genetic basis of FMD is understood incompletely. Genetic variants can be sporadic or familial, and only a minority of patients (1.9%–7.3%) with FMD report an affected family member.[20] Genetic screening for FMD is currently not supported nor are associated variants considered actionable by the American College of Medical Genetics.[22]

Several clinical findings suggest RVD as the underlying cause of hypertension. The American College of Cardiology/American Heart Association guidelines suggest screening for RVD among patients with (1) resistant hypertension, (2) abrupt onset hypertension, (3) hypertension that is increasingly difficult to control, especially in the context of flash pulmonary edema, and (4) early-onset hypertension (especially in females, given risk of FMD).[2] The 2018 European Society of Cardiology/European Society of Hypertension (ESH) hypertension guidelines also describe signs and symptoms suggestive of RVD, which include widespread atherosclerosis (especially peripheral arterial disease), diabetes, smoking, recurrent flash pulmonary edema, and abdominal bruit.[23] The ESH and the Society for Vascular Medicine note that FMD should be considered in those with (1) an onset of hypertension at less than 30 years of age, (2) accelerated and/or malignant hypertension (>180/110), (3) drug resistance, (4) unilateral small kidney without causative urologic abnormality, (5) abdominal bruit in the absence of atherosclerotic risk factors, (6) suspected renal artery dissection, or (7) the presence of FMD in another artery.[24]

Screening for RVD should be performed when patients have evidence of secondary hypertension without other obvious secondary causes and when an intervention would likely be planned if a significant stenotic lesion is found. Testing is generally not performed in patients who are well-controlled with medical therapy. The gold standard for diagnosing RVD is renal angiogram. Although a renal angiogram is invasive and involves the use of radiocontrast dye, it allows for relatively precise measurement of flow gradients, which can discern clinically significant lesions. Alternative modalities include renal duplex Doppler ultrasound examination, magnetic resonance angiography, and CT angiography.[2] The choice of screening test is based on institutional factors (local expertise, availability) and patient factors (renal function, allergies, body habitus, preference).

Generally, noninvasive imaging is considered less reliable than a renal angiogram for the diagnosis of FMD. Duplex Doppler ultrasound examination is widely available and inexpensive, but technical expertise is center dependent.[25] The ESH/Society for Vascular Medicine consensus group recommends CTA as the initial screening test when FMD is suspected, or magnetic resonance angiography if CT angiography is contraindicated. Per the ESH/Society for Vascular Medicine, CT angiography is preferable to magnetic resonance angiography for the diagnosis of FMD because of superior spatial resolution and better discrimination of FMD from atherosclerotic RVD.[24]

There are 3 treatment categories for RVD: (1) medical, (2) angioplasty with or without stenting, and (3) surgical. Medical therapy is the first-line treatment in all cases of RVD. The European Society of Cardiology and American Heart Association recommend angiotensin-converting enzyme inhibitor, angiotensin-receptor blocker, or calcium channel blocker therapy, with a specific recommendation from the European Society of Cardiology to closely monitor the estimated glomerular filtration rate and potassium upon initiation of an angiotensin-converting enzyme inhibitor/angiotensin-receptor blocker.[2,26] Although angiotensin-converting enzyme inhibitors and angiotensin-receptor blockers are generally well-tolerated, a decreased in the estimated glomerular filtration rate of more than 30% may prompt consideration of renal revascularization. Other important aspects of medical management of RVD include optimal management of hypercholesterolemia, diabetes mellitus, and obesity; tobacco cessation; and the use of an antiplatelet agent.

The role of renal angioplasty with or without stenting remains controversial in atherosclerotic RVD but is accepted in FMD. Based on a 2014 Cochrane systematic review of 8 randomized controlled trials involving 2222 participants, angioplasty with or without stenting was not shown to be superior to medical therapy in atherosclerotic RVD.[27] Surgical treatment of RVD is less common given the emphasis on medical therapy and the availability of percutaneous intervention. Generally, surgical revascularization or bypass is considered in patients with anatomically complex disease refractory to medical management or those undergoing vascular repair for other reasons.

Obstructive Sleep Apnea

OSA is a breathing disorder where the upper airway recurrently collapses during sleep and induces intermittent hypoxemia.[28] Several studies have established a strong and consistent association between OSA and hypertension. In a systematic review and meta-analysis evaluating this association, Hou and colleagues[29] examined 26 studies that included more than 50,000 participants and demonstrated that OSA is significantly associated with both essential and primary and resistant hypertension. Furthermore, episodes of apnea are significant predictors of both systolic and diastolic blood pressure; each episode of apnea per hour of sleep is associated with a 1% increased odds of hypertension.[30] A dose–response relationship has been established, wherein the risk of hypertension increases linearly with increasing severity of OSA.[30,31] Furthermore, OSA has been found in more than 80% of patients with resistant hypertension,[32,33] with the greatest prevalence among those with refractory hypertension.[34]

The risk of acquiring OSA is influenced by several modifiable and unmodifiable risk factors. Unmodifiable risk factors include advancing age, male sex, craniofacial anatomy, and family history of OSA. Modifiable risk factors include smoking, alcohol use, nasal congestion, and, most commonly, obesity.[35,36] There is a strong, direct correlation between obesity and OSA; a 10% increase in body weight is associated with a 6-fold increased risk of having OSA.[37]

Screening for OSA should be considered in patients reporting sleep problems such as breathing pauses at night, snoring, and excessive daytime sleepiness or fatigue.[38] Screening for OSA should also be considered in individuals with known risk factors as well as those with comorbidities that may be attributed to OSA, such as resistant hypertension, heart failure, arrythmias, coronary artery disease, and stroke, as well as metabolic disorders including diabetes, glucose intolerance, and hyperlipidemia.[39–41] Several brief questionnaires are used for risk assessment such as the Berlin questionnaire or Epworth Sleepiness Scale, but the most accurate remains the STOP-Bang questionnaire.[42–44] Ultimately, the gold standard test to establish the diagnosis is laboratory-based polysomnography, where both respiratory and sleep parameters are monitored.[45]

The treatment of OSA carries several benefits, including improvement in blood pressure. Several treatment modalities are available including behavioral measures such as avoidance of tobacco and alcohol and adjusting sleep positioning, medical devices such as mandibular repositioning appliances, or surgical procedures such as uvulopalatopharyngoplasty or maxillomandibular advancement.[38] The mainstays of treatment, however, are continuous positive airway pressure (CPAP) and medically supervised weight loss. The use of CPAP for treatment of OSA is associated with improvements in blood pressure, with varying results depending on the severity of hypertension. In patients with moderate hypertension, the use of CPAP is associated with a modest decrease in the systolic blood pressure and diastolic blood pressure (mean decrease of 3 mm Hg and 2 mm Hg, respectively) in addition to an improvement in blood pressure variability.[46–48] The antihypertensive effect of CPAP therapy is greater in patients with resistant hypertension (mean decrease of 6–7 mm Hg systolic blood pressure and 4–5 mm Hg diastolic blood pressure).[49,50] Data also support that the treatment of OSA with weight loss can have a significant effect on blood pressure. Surgical weight loss is associated with lower OSA severity and remission of hypertension in a subset of patients.[51,52] The most robust improvement in blood pressure, however, can be achieved when CPAP is used in conjunction with weight loss. In a randomized controlled trial, Chirinos and colleagues[53] assessed the antihypertensive effect of weight loss and CPAP use both alone and in combination. The authors found a decrease in the systolic blood pressure of 6.8 mm Hg with weight loss, 3.0 mm Hg with CPAP use, and 14.1 mm Hg in the dual intervention group. This finding suggests that the treatment of OSA with combined weight loss and CPAP can have a synergistic effect on blood pressure control.

MEDICATION-, DRUG-, AND ALCOHOL-INDUCED HYPERTENSION

Prescription medications, over-the-counter medications and supplements, illicit drugs, and alcohol are common causes of secondary hypertension.[54] A careful history is necessary to determine patients' risks of hypertension owing to prescribed or non-prescribed substances, including illicit drug use.[55,56] Serum or urine screening for toxins may be appropriate in some patients. Ideally, in patients with hypertension, and particularly those with resistant hypertension, drugs that increase blood pressure should be discontinued in lieu of alternative agents that do not affect blood pressure.

Examples of drugs that can increase blood pressure are outlined in **Table 2**, including recommendations for addressing the use of these agents and alternative therapies. Some examples are highlighted here. Drugs prescribed for psychiatric conditions, including attention deficit hyperactivity disorder, depression, and psychosis, are commonly associated with increased blood pressure. Providers should evaluate the appropriateness of recommending alternative approaches, such as behavioral therapy or medications that do not generally affect blood pressure (eg, selective serotonin reuptake inhibitors, aripiprazole, and ziprasidone).[2,57] Several chemotherapeutic agents increase blood pressure, including anti-vascular endothelial growth factor therapy, tyrosine kinase inhibitors, and alkylating agents. These medications should generally be continued, and their use should be accompanied by very close monitoring of blood pressure and anticipated escalation of antihypertensive therapy.[58] Of note, sudden withdrawal of centrally acting alpha-agonists, such as clonidine (commonly used as an antihypertensive medication) and tizanidine (increasingly used as a muscle relaxant) can result in severe rebound hypertension.[59,60] These medications should ideally be avoided in patients with hypertension owing to this risk; if they are used, they should be tapered slowly upon cessation.

Nonsteroidal anti-inflammatory drugs are associated with a modest increase in blood pressure, the development of new onset hypertension, and worsening blood pressure control among patients already diagnosed with hypertension.[61–63] Some patients require escalation of antihypertensive therapy to counter these effects. Where possible, alternative agents should be used, particularly among patients with resistant hypertension. If nonsteroidal anti-inflammatory agents are necessary, blood pressure should be monitoring closely and antihypertensive therapy should be escalated as needed, preferentially using non–renin-angiotensin-aldosterone system–inhibiting agents.[64,65]

Alcohol intake is associated with increased blood pressure and an increased risk of developing hypertension, particularly heavy alcohol intake of 3 or more standard drinks per day (>36 oz of beer, 15 oz of wine, or 4.5 ounces of spirits).[2,66] In the United States, excess alcohol intake is thought to contribute to up to 10% of cases of hypertension. A decrease in alcohol intake by about 50% among heavy drinkers lowers blood pressure by a mean of 5/4 mm Hg in randomized controlled trials.[67,68] Current hypertension guidelines recommend that women drink no more than 1 standard drink and men drink no more than 2 standard drinks daily.[2]

PHEOCHROMOCYTOMA AND PARAGANGLIOMA

Pheochromocytomas are rare catecholamine-secreting tumors of the adrenal gland. In approximately 10% of cases, these tumors occur in extra-adrenal locations that are derived from sympathetic or parasympathetic nerves, called paragangliomas. Pheochromocytomas occur in as few of 0.01% to 0.20% of patients with hypertension, with a higher prevalence in those with resistant hypertension.[69] These tumors are often accompanied by paroxysmal hypertension and tachycardia as well as other

Table 2
Prescription and nonprescription drugs that increase blood pressure and alternative approaches

Drugs that Increase Blood Pressure	Alternative Approaches in Patients with Hypertension
Prescription drugs	
Amphetamines	Recommend behavioral therapy[73]
Antidepressants, including monoamine oxidase inhibitors, serotonin norepinephrine reuptake inhibitors, norepinephrine and dopamine reuptake inhibitors, and tricyclic antidepressants	Recommend alternative antidepressants including selective serotonin reuptake inhibitors[54]
Atypical antipsychotics including clozapine and olanzapine	Recommend alternative atypical antipsychotics such as aripiprazole and ziprasidone[2,57]
Immunosuppressing medications including cyclosporine and systemic corticosteroids	Recommend alternative immunosuppressing medications including tacrolimus and mycophenolate[74]
Estradiol-containing oral contraceptives	Recommend progestin-only contraceptives or alternative forms of contraception
Chemotherapeutic agents including anti- vascular endothelial growth factor therapy, tyrosine kinase inhibitors, and alkylating agents	Typically recommend close monitoring of blood pressure and escalation of antihypertensive therapy[58]
Sudden withdrawal of central-acting sympatholytic drugs such as clonidine and tizanidine	Recommend avoiding oral clonidine for treatment of hypertension whenever possible and tapering upon discontinuation[59]; use cyclobenzaprine or other muscle relaxants instead of tizanidine[60]
Nonprescription drugs	
Alcohol	Recommend limiting use to no more than 1 drink/d in women and 2 drinks/d in men[2]
Caffeine	Recommend limiting use to <300 mg/d[2,75]
Cocaine	Recommend abstinence
Methamphetamine	Recommend abstinence
Decongestants that include pseudoephedrine or phenylephrine	Decongestants such as antihistamines
Supplements such as ephedra and St. John's wort	Recommend abstinence[76]
Nonsteroidal anti-inflammatory drugs	Acetaminophen or topical nonsteroidal agents

symptoms, including piloerection, headache, and palpitations.[70] Thus, an evaluation for pheochromocytoma is typically reserved for patients with paroxysmal hypertension and/or symptomatic hypertension. Testing for pheochromocytoma should include either plasma (preferable owing to the ease of assessment) or 24-hour urine metanephrines. These tests can be elevated in primary hypertension, obesity, and

OSA, but have high sensitivity and specificity for pheochromocytoma or paraganglioma at higher levels, typically 2.5- to 3.0-fold higher than the upper limit of normal.[69,71] Patients with significantly elevated metanephrines should undergo a CT scan to localize the tumor (or alternatively an MRI) and metaiodobenzylguanidine scanning to evaluate for metastases.[70] Furthermore, because approximately one-third of cases are inherited, patients should undergo genetic testing. The mainstay of treatment for pheochromocytoma is surgical resection, where feasible, with preoperative alpha-blockade to prevent blood pressure instability and postoperative monitoring for recurrence and metastases.[70]

ADDITIONAL RARE CAUSES OF SECONDARY HYPERTENSION

There are several additional rare causes of secondary hypertension that each occur in less than 1% of patients with hypertension, such as Cushing syndrome, hypothyroidism, hyperthyroidism, coarctation of the aorta, primary hyperparathyroidism, and acromegaly.[2,69] Given its relatively high prevalence in the general population, assessment for thyroid disease with a thyroid-stimulating hormone test is generally recommended as part of the initial evaluation for hypertension; however, hypertension typically only occurs as a result of severe forms of thyroid disease and merits treatment regardless of thyroid hormone levels.[72] Similarly, primary hyperparathyroidism should be suspected in individuals with concomitant hypertension and hypercalcemia. Given their infrequency, patients should only be assessed for the remaining rare etiologies of secondary hypertension based on specific historical and examination findings. For example, Cushing's syndrome occurs in less than 0.1% of patients with hypertension, and typically presents with systemic evidence of cortisol excess besides hypertension, including central obesity after rapid weight gain, hyperglycemia, proximal muscle weakness, striae, and hirsutism.

SUMMARY

Secondary hypertension is common among patients with hypertension and is often underrecognized. Furthermore, secondary hypertension can result in target organ damage independent of the effects of blood pressure alone, which can be mitigated with appropriate management. Patients with hypertension should be evaluated for risk factors for secondary hypertension and screened accordingly. In particular, patients with resistant hypertension should, at a minimum, undergo testing for PA and screening for drugs that may induce hypertension, with further evaluation for renovascular hypertension and OSA depending on their age, symptoms, and comorbidities. Rarer causes of secondary hypertension should be considered depending on the clinical picture. Given the high prevalence of hypertension in the general population, greater attention is needed to identify causes of secondary hypertension, which can be pivotal to improving blood pressure control and preventing cardiovascular events in these high-risk patients.

CLINICS CARE POINTS

- Patients with hypertension can benefit from evaluation for secondary hypertension to decrease the risk of refractory hypertension and target organ damage independent of blood pressure control.
- Patients with an early age of onset of hypertension and resistant hypertension, in particular, should undergo evaluation for secondary hypertension.

- Provider history taking is critical to assessing patients for secondary hypertension, particularly the identification of risk factors for secondary hypertension.
- All patients with hypertension should be screened for use of prescription and nonprescription drugs that may increase blood pressure and whether alternative therapies may be appropriate.

DISCLOSURE

All authors report no relevant disclosures. Dr J.B. Cohen is supported by the National Institutes of Health National Heart, Lung, and Blood Institute K23-HL133843 and R01-HL153646, National Center for Advancing Translational Sciences U01-TR003734, National Institute of Diabetes and Digestive and Kidney Diseases R01-DK123104and U24-DK060990 and American Heart Association Bugher Award.

REFERENCES

1. Mills KT, Bundy JD, Kelly TN, et al. Global disparities of hypertension prevalence and control: a systematic analysis of population-based studies From 90 Countries. Circulation 2016;134(6):441–50.
2. Whelton PK, Carey RM, Aronow WS, et al. 2017 ACC/AHA/AAPA/ABC/ACPM/AGS/APhA/ASH/ASPC/NMA/PCNA guideline for the prevention, detection, evaluation, and management of high blood pressure in adults: a report of the American College of Cardiology/American Heart Association Task Force on Clinical Practice Guidelines. Hypertension 2018;71(6):e13–115.
3. Byrd JB, Turcu AF, Auchus RJ. Primary aldosteronism: practical approach to diagnosis and management. Circulation 2018;138(8):823–35.
4. Monticone S, D'Ascenzo F, Moretti C, et al. Cardiovascular events and target organ damage in primary aldosteronism compared with essential hypertension: a systematic review and meta-analysis. Lancet Diabetes Endocrinol 2018;6(1):41–50.
5. Funder JW, Carey RM, Mantero F, et al. The management of primary aldosteronism: case detection, diagnosis, and treatment: an Endocrine Society Clinical Practice Guideline. J Clin Endocrinol Metab 2016;101(5):1889–916.
6. Brown JM, Robinson-Cohen C, Luque-Fernandez MA, et al. The spectrum of subclinical primary aldosteronism and incident hypertension: a cohort study. Ann Intern Med 2017;167(9):630–41.
7. Monticone S, Burrello J, Tizzani D, et al. Prevalence and clinical manifestations of primary aldosteronism encountered in primary care practice. J Am Coll Cardiol 2017;69(14):1811–20.
8. Kayser SC, Dekkers T, Groenewoud HJ, et al. Study heterogeneity and estimation of prevalence of primary aldosteronism: a systematic review and meta-regression analysis. J Clin Endocrinol Metab 2016;101(7):2826–35.
9. Jaffe G, Gray Z, Krishnan G, et al. Screening rates for primary aldosteronism in resistant hypertension: a cohort study. Hypertension 2020;75(3):650–9.
10. Cohen JB, Cohen DL, Herman DS, et al. Testing for primary aldosteronism and mineralocorticoid receptor antagonist use among U.S. Veterans: a retrospective cohort study. Ann Intern Med 2021;174(3):289–97.
11. Brown JM, Siddiqui M, Calhoun DA, et al. The unrecognized prevalence of primary aldosteronism. Ann Intern Med 2020;173(1):10–20.

12. Jakobsson H, Farmaki K, Sakinis A, et al. Adrenal venous sampling: the learning curve of a single interventionalist with 282 consecutive procedures. Diagn Interv Radiol 2018;24(2):89–93.

13. Chrysochou C, Kalra PA. Epidemiology and natural history of atherosclerotic renovascular disease. Prog Cardiovasc Dis 2009;52(3):184–95.

14. Hansen KJ, Edwards MS, Craven TE, et al. Prevalence of renovascular disease in the elderly: a population-based study. J Vasc Surg 2002;36(3):443–51.

15. Safian RD, Textor SC. Renal-artery stenosis. N Engl J Med 2001;344(6):431–42.

16. Krijnen P, van Jaarsveld BC, Steyerberg EW, et al. A clinical prediction rule for renal artery stenosis. Ann Intern Med 1998;129(9):705–11.

17. Herrmann SM, Textor SC. Renovascular hypertension. Endocrinol Metab Clin North Am 2019;48(4):765–78.

18. Libby P, Buring JE, Badimon L, et al. Atherosclerosis. Nat Rev Dis Primers 2019; 5(1):56.

19. Plouin PF, Baguet JP, Thony F, et al. High prevalence of multiple arterial bed lesions in patients with fibromuscular dysplasia: the ARCADIA Registry (Assessment of Renal and Cervical Artery Dysplasia). Hypertension 2017;70(3):652–8.

20. Olin JW, Froehlich J, Gu X, et al. The United States Registry for Fibromuscular Dysplasia: results in the first 447 patients. Circulation 2012;125(25):3182–90.

21. Perdu J, Boutouyrie P, Bourgain C, et al. Inheritance of arterial lesions in renal fibromuscular dysplasia. J Hum Hypertens 2007;21(5):393–400.

22. Kalia SS, Adelman K, Bale SJ, et al. Recommendations for reporting of secondary findings in clinical exome and genome sequencing, 2016 update (ACMG SF v2.0): a policy statement of the American College of Medical Genetics and Genomics. Genet Med 2017;19(2):249–55.

23. Williams B, Mancia G, Spiering W, et al. 2018 ESC/ESH Guidelines for the management of arterial hypertension. Eur Heart J 2018;39(33):3021–104.

24. Gornik HL, Persu A, Adlam D, et al. First international consensus on the diagnosis and management of fibromuscular dysplasia. J Hypertens 2019;37(2):229–52.

25. Williams GJ, Macaskill P, Chan SF, et al. Comparative accuracy of renal duplex sonographic parameters in the diagnosis of renal artery stenosis: paired and unpaired analysis. AJR Am J Roentgenol 2007;188(3):798–811.

26. Aboyans V, Ricco JB, Bartelink MEL, et al. 2017 ESC Guidelines on the Diagnosis and Treatment of Peripheral Arterial Diseases, in collaboration with the European Society for Vascular Surgery (ESVS): document covering atherosclerotic disease of extracranial carotid and vertebral, mesenteric, renal, upper and lower extremity arteries. Endorsed by: the European Stroke Organization (ESO), The Task Force for the Diagnosis and Treatment of Peripheral Arterial Diseases of the European Society of Cardiology (ESC) and of the European Society for Vascular Surgery (ESVS). Eur Heart J 2018;39(9):763–816.

27. Jenks S, Yeoh SE, Conway BR. Balloon angioplasty, with and without stenting, versus medical therapy for hypertensive patients with renal artery stenosis. Cochrane Database Syst Rev 2014;2014(12):CD002944.

28. Patel SR. Obstructive sleep apnea. Ann Intern Med 2019;171(11):itc81–96.

29. Hou H, Zhao Y, Yu W, et al. Association of obstructive sleep apnea with hypertension: a systematic review and meta-analysis. J Glob Health 2018;8(1):010405.

30. Lavie P, Herer P, Hoffstein V. Obstructive sleep apnoea syndrome as a risk factor for hypertension: population study. BMJ 2000;320(7233):479–82.

31. Young T, Peppard P, Palta M, et al. Population-based study of sleep-disordered breathing as a risk factor for hypertension. Arch Intern Med 1997;157(15): 1746–52.

32. Pedrosa RP, Drager LF, Gonzaga CC, et al. Obstructive sleep apnea. Hypertension 2011;58(5):811–7.

33. Muxfeldt ES, Margallo VS, Guimarães GM, et al. Prevalence and associated factors of obstructive sleep apnea in patients with resistant hypertension. Am J Hypertens 2014;27(8):1069–78.

34. Martínez-García M-A, Navarro-Soriano C, Torres G, et al. Beyond resistant hypertension. Hypertension 2018;72(3):618–24.

35. Rundo JV. Obstructive sleep apnea basics. Cleve Clin J Med 2019;86(9 Suppl 1):2–9.

36. Abu Salman L, Shulman R, Cohen JB. Obstructive sleep apnea, hypertension, and cardiovascular risk: epidemiology, pathophysiology, and management. Curr Cardiol Rep 2020;22(2):6.

37. Peppard PE, Young T, Palta M, et al. Longitudinal study of moderate weight change and sleep-disordered breathing. JAMA 2000;284(23):3015–21.

38. Gottlieb DJ, Punjabi NM. Diagnosis and management of obstructive sleep apnea: a review. JAMA 2020;323(14):1389–400.

39. Javaheri S, Barbe F, Campos-Rodriguez F, et al. Sleep Apnea. J Am Coll Cardiol 2017;69(7):841–58.

40. Strausz S, Havulinna AS, Tuomi T, et al. Obstructive sleep apnoea and the risk for coronary heart disease and type 2 diabetes: a longitudinal population-based study in Finland. BMJ Open 2018;8(10):e022752.

41. Nadeem R, Singh M, Nida M, et al. Effect of obstructive sleep apnea hypopnea syndrome on lipid profile: a meta-regression analysis. J Clin Sleep Med 2014; 10(5):475–89.

42. Netzer NC, Stoohs RA, Netzer CM, et al. Using the Berlin Questionnaire to identify patients at risk for the sleep apnea syndrome. Ann Intern Med 1999;131(7): 485–91.

43. Chung F, Yegneswaran B, Liao P, et al. STOP questionnaire: a tool to screen patients for obstructive sleep apnea. Anesthesiology 2008;108(5):812–21.

44. Chiu HY, Chen PY, Chuang LP, et al. Diagnostic accuracy of the Berlin questionnaire, STOP-BANG, STOP, and Epworth sleepiness scale in detecting obstructive sleep apnea: a bivariate meta-analysis. Sleep Med Rev 2017;36:57–70.

45. Kapur VK, Auckley DH, Chowdhuri S, et al. Clinical practice guideline for diagnostic testing for adult obstructive sleep apnea: an American Academy of Sleep Medicine Clinical Practice Guideline. J Clin Sleep Med 2017;13(3):479–504.

46. Pengo MF, Ratneswaran C, Berry M, et al. Effect of continuous positive airway pressure on blood pressure variability in patients with obstructive sleep apnea. J Clin Hypertens 2016;18(11):1180–4.

47. Bazzano LA, Khan Z, Reynolds K, et al. Effect of nocturnal nasal continuous positive airway pressure on blood pressure in obstructive sleep apnea. Hypertension 2007;50(2):417–23.

48. Hu X, Fan J, Chen S, et al. The role of continuous positive airway pressure in blood pressure control for patients with obstructive sleep apnea and hypertension: a meta-analysis of randomized controlled trials. J Clin Hypertens 2015; 17(3):215–22.

49. Iftikhar IH, Valentine CW, Bittencourt LR, et al. Effects of continuous positive airway pressure on blood pressure in patients with resistant hypertension and obstructive sleep apnea: a meta-analysis. J Hypertens 2014;32(12):2341–50 [discussion: 2350].

50. Pedrosa RP, Drager LF, de Paula LKG, et al. Effects of OSA treatment on BP in patients with resistant hypertension: a randomized trial. Chest 2013;144(5): 1487–94.

51. Cohen JB, Cohen DL. Cardiovascular and renal effects of weight reduction in obesity and the metabolic syndrome. Curr Hypertens Rep 2015;17(5):34.

52. Peromaa-Haavisto P, Tuomilehto H, Kössi J, et al. Obstructive sleep apnea: the effect of bariatric surgery after 12 months. A prospective multicenter trial. Sleep Med 2017;35:85–90.

53. Chirinos JA, Gurubhagavatula I, Teff K, et al. CPAP, weight loss, or both for obstructive sleep apnea. N Engl J Med 2014;370(24):2265–75.

54. Foy MC, Vaishnav J, Sperati CJ. Drug-induced hypertension. Endocrinol Metab Clin North Am 2019;48(4):859–73.

55. Goldstein LB, Bushnell CD, Adams RJ, et al. Guidelines for the primary prevention of stroke: a guideline for healthcare professionals from the American Heart Association/American Stroke Association. Stroke 2011;42(2):517–84.

56. Cohen JB, Townsend RR. Evaluation of hypertension. Nephrol Self-Assessment Program 2020;19(1):8–19.

57. Newcomer JW. Metabolic considerations in the use of antipsychotic medications: a review of recent evidence. J Clin Psychiatry 2007;68(Suppl 1):20–7.

58. Cohen JB, Geara AS, Hogan JJ, et al. Hypertension in cancer patients and survivors: epidemiology, diagnosis, and management. JACC CardioOncol 2019; 1(2):238–51.

59. Geyskes GG, Boer P, Dorhout Mees EJ. Clonidine withdrawal. Mechanism and frequency of rebound hypertension. Br J Clin Pharmacol 1979;7(1):55–62.

60. Luther JM, Dominiczak AF, Jennings GLR, et al. Paroxysmal hypertension associated with presyncope. Hypertension 2019;74(4):718–25.

61. Yang M, Wang HT, Zhao M, et al. Network meta-analysis comparing relatively selective COX-2 inhibitors versus coxibs for the prevention of NSAID-induced gastrointestinal injury. Medicine (Baltimore) 2015;94(40):e1592.

62. Aw TJ, Haas SJ, Liew D, et al. Meta-analysis of cyclooxygenase-2 inhibitors and their effects on blood pressure. Arch Intern Med 2005;165(5):490–6.

63. Chan CC, Reid CM, Aw TJ, et al. Do COX-2 inhibitors raise blood pressure more than nonselective NSAIDs and placebo? An updated meta-analysis. J Hypertens 2009;27(12):2332–41.

64. Szeto CC, Sugano K, Wang JG, et al. Non-steroidal anti-inflammatory drug (NSAID) therapy in patients with hypertension, cardiovascular, renal or gastrointestinal comorbidities: joint APAGE/APLAR/APSDE/APSH/APSN/PoA recommendations. Gut 2020;69(4):617–29.

65. Dreischulte T, Morales DR, Bell S, et al. Combined use of nonsteroidal anti-inflammatory drugs with diuretics and/or renin-angiotensin system inhibitors in the community increases the risk of acute kidney injury. Kidney Int 2015;88(2): 396–403.

66. Klatsky AL. Alcohol and cardiovascular mortality: common sense and scientific truth. J Am Coll Cardiol 2010;55(13):1336–8.

67. Xin X, He J, Frontini MG, et al. Effects of alcohol reduction on blood pressure: a meta-analysis of randomized controlled trials. Hypertension 2001;38(5):1112–7.

68. Roerecke M, Kaczorowski J, Tobe SW, et al. The effect of a reduction in alcohol consumption on blood pressure: a systematic review and meta-analysis. Lancet Public Health 2017;2(2):e108–20.

69. Carey RM, Calhoun DA, Bakris GL, et al. Resistant hypertension: detection, evaluation, and management: a scientific statement from the American Heart Association. Hypertension 2018;72(5):e53–90.
70. Lenders JW, Duh QY, Eisenhofer G, et al. Pheochromocytoma and paraganglioma: an endocrine society clinical practice guideline. J Clin Endocrinol Metab 2014;99(6):1915–42.
71. Schwartz GL. Screening for adrenal-endocrine hypertension: overview of accuracy and cost-effectiveness. Endocrinol Metab Clin North Am 2011;40(2): 279–94, vii.
72. Hofstetter L, Messerli FH. Hypothyroidism and hypertension: fact or myth? Lancet 2018;391(10115):29–30.
73. Cortese S, Holtmann M, Banaschewski T, et al. Practitioner review: current best practice in the management of adverse events during treatment with ADHD medications in children and adolescents. J Child Psychol Psychiatry 2013;54(3): 227–46.
74. Xue W, Zhang Q, Xu Y, et al. Effects of tacrolimus and cyclosporine treatment on metabolic syndrome and cardiovascular risk factors after renal transplantation: a meta-analysis. Chin Med J (Engl) 2014;127(12):2376–81.
75. Mesas AE, Leon-Munoz LM, Rodriguez-Artalejo F, et al. The effect of coffee on blood pressure and cardiovascular disease in hypertensive individuals: a systematic review and meta-analysis. Am J Clin Nutr 2011;94(4):1113–26.
76. Tachjian A, Maria V, Jahangir A. Use of herbal products and potential interactions in patients with cardiovascular diseases. J Am Coll Cardiol 2010;55(6):515–25.

What is the Optimal Low-Density Lipoprotein Cholesterol?

Andrew Gagel, MD[a], Fawzi Zghyer, MD[a], Christeen Samuel[b], Seth S. Martin, MD, MHS[c,d],*

KEYWORDS

- Low-density lipoprotein cholesterol (LDL-C)
- Atherosclerotic cardiovascular disease (ASCVD) • Cerebrovascular accident (CVA)
- Peripheral arterial disease (PAD)

KEY POINTS

- Long-term exposure to lower low-density lipoprotein cholesterol (LDL-C) levels is associated with a lower risk of cardiovascular events compared with shorter term exposure to lower LDL-C.
- Cardiovascular prevention should target cumulative exposure to LDL-C by aiming to lower LDL-C earlier in life.
- The cardioprotective impact of lipid-lowering therapies extends to very low LDL-C levels (10 mg/dL) with no known cardiovascular benefit plateau.
- There is no known lower limit with respect to safety when treating LDL-C in high-risk patients.

INTRODUCTION

Low-density lipoprotein cholesterol (LDL-C) is a well-established, causal factor for atherosclerotic cardiovascular disease (ASCVD). Mendelian randomization studies have demonstrated that long-term exposure to lower LDL-C levels is associated with a lower risk of cardiovascular events compared with shorter-term exposure to lower LDL-C.[1] The clinical benefit of lowering LDL-C with statins is widely accepted as is the concept that the magnitude of clinical benefit observed with statins is

[a] Johns Hopkins University School of Medicine, 1830 E Monument Street, Baltimore, MD 21287, USA; [b] Johns Hopkins University School of Medicine, 733 North Broadway, Baltimore, MD 21205, USA; [c] Johns Hopkins University School of Medicine, Johns Hopkins Hospital, 600 North Wolfe Street, Carnegie 591, Baltimore, MD 21287, USA; [d] Advanced Lipid Disorders Program, Ciccarone Center for the Prevention of Cardiovascular Disease, 600 North Wolfe Street, Carnegie 591, Baltimore, MD 21287, USA
* Corresponding author. Johns Hopkins Hospital, 600 North Wolfe Street, Carnegie 591, Baltimore, MD 21287.
E-mail address: smart100@jhmi.edu
Twitter: @SethShayMartin (S.S.M.)

Med Clin N Am 106 (2022) 285–298
https://doi.org/10.1016/j.mcna.2021.11.005
medical.theclinics.com
0025-7125/22/© 2021 Elsevier Inc. All rights reserved.

proportional to the absolute reduction in LDL-C.[2–5] Yet, in an era of nonstatin drugs (eg, ezetimibe and proprotein convertase subtilisin/kexin type 9 [PCSK9] inhibitors) that can lower LDL-C levels to unprecedented levels, uncertainty remains regarding the optimal approach toward lowering LDL-C: which patients should be treated with which lipid-lowering therapies, when should therapy be started, and how low should we go with LDL-C? This article aims to review the current data on the effects of lowering LDL-C and give insight to the clinician on how to effectively reduce ASCVD risk.

BACKGROUND: LIPID METABOLISM AND SYNTHESIS

The exogenous pathway of lipid metabolism begins in the stomach where gastric and pancreatic lipases hydrolyze ingested lipids. In the intestinal tract, bile acids and lipids form biliary micelles that are absorbed by intestinal villi. The Niemann-Pick C1-like 1 protein, the target of ezetimibe, facilitates transport of micelles into enterocytes. Other transport proteins, as CD36, aid in the absorption of deesterified fatty acids and monoacylglycerols. Absorbed cholesterol and triglycerides are assembled into chylomicrons via pathways that rely on microsomal triglyceride transfer protein and $ApoB_{48}$. Chylomicrons are then secreted into the intestinal lymphatic system and subsequently into the bloodstream.[6]

Hepatic synthesis of cholesterol begins through conversion of glucose to pyruvate via acetyl CoA. B-hydroxy B-methylglutaryl-CoA reductase, the target for statins, through multiple intermediates, forms cholesterols. Microsomal triglyceride transfer protein then joins triglyceride with cholesterol, cholesteryl ester, phospholipid, and $Apo-B_{100}$, to assemble into particles of very-low-density lipoproteins (VLDLs) that eventually make it into the bloodstream. High-density lipoprotein (HDL) is formed by the efflux of cholesterol and phospholipids from the liver by means of ATP-binding cassette transporter A1 into apolipoprotein A-I or smaller HDLs.

Chylomicrons and VLDLs undergo lipolysis by lipoprotein lipase, becoming a source of energy for muscle cells. Unused chylomicrons and VLDLs are stored in adipocytes, forming chylomicron and VLDL remnants, which later form LDL-C. Circulating LDL-C is cleared from the bloodstream by hepatic LDL receptors, which in turn are broken down by PCSK9. Atherogenesis occurs when ApoB-containing particles deposit in the arterial wall after undergoing oxidation. Those particles are then internalized by macrophages and create foam cells and eventually plaques.[6]

BACKGROUND: LOW-DENSITY LIPOPROTEIN CHOLESTEROL MEASUREMENT

Given the importance of LDL-C in prevention, its accurate measurement is paramount. Past LDL-C measurement methods used in clinical settings were accurate in the average patient but unreliable in individuals with dyslipidemia, diabetes mellitus, and/or metabolic disorders.[7,8] The field has since sought to leverage adjustable formulas to better account for variance among patients. Current methods of measuring LDL-C include (1) preparative ultracentrifuge (PUC), (2) homogeneous detergent-based automated LDL-C assays or direct assays, and (3) calculation-based measurements (**Table 1**).

PUC is the gold standard for LDL-C assessment; however, it is a laborious, high-cost technique that is primarily used as a reference standard in research settings. Other nonultracentrifuge, chemical-based direct assays that use detergents and other chemicals to obtain targeted blocking or solubilization of lipoprotein classes have emerged but with drawbacks.[8] Their variable, nonstandardized techniques and limited data supporting their accuracy lead to method-dependent differences in LDL-C and

Table 1
A comparison of methods to determine patient's low-density lipoprotein cholesterol level

Method	Strengths	Limitations	Availability
Ultracentrifugation	Gold standard	Tedious High cost	Research settings
Friedewald equation	Low cost Widely validated Reliable in most of the patients	Inaccurate at high triglycerides (TG) (2.0–4.5 mmol/L) Underestimates LDL-C in high-risk patients	Clinical laboratories
Martin/Hopkins equation	Low cost Widely validated Reliable in most of the patients Accurate at high TG Accurate at low LDL-C Accurate in nonfasting states	Inaccurate at very high TG (>4.5 mmol/L)	Johns Hopkins Quest diagnostics Other laboratories
Direct LDL-C assays	Accurate at TG > 4.5 mmol/L	Not well validated Not reliable in most of the patients Not standardized	Clinically available

could complicate longitudinal patient management.[9] Because direct assay methods still lack widely validated clinical and financial advantages in performance, they are unlikely to surpass calculation-based methods that are currently entrenched in routine practice.[8]

Two main equations, the Friedewald equation and the Martin/Hopkins equation, have emerged as cost-effective methods of measuring LDL-C. Before publication of the novel Martin/Hopkins equation in 2013, the Friedewald equation was the method of choice by many clinical laboratories. However, the Friedewald equation has significant limitations arising from its use of a fixed conversion factor in calculating LDL-C levels, leading to increasingly inaccurate results at low LDL-C and high triglyceride levels (as commonly seen in patients with diabetes and renal disease).[8]

An influx of new equations modified the original Friedewald formula, but most were only appropriate in particular subsets of the population or failed to provide independent validation against reference standards. In 2013, Martin and colleagues developed an equation with a similar structure as Friedewald but using distinct, adjustable factors based on individuals' triglyceride and non–HDL-C levels.[10] The equation was derived from a representative population of 1,350,000 patients from the Very Large Database of Lipids Study and was independently validated on an international level.[11,12] Importantly, the Martin/Hopkins method has subsequently been validated in different segments of the patient population, including patients on PCSK9 inhibitors,[12] patients with diabetes,[13] patients with familial combined hyperlipidemia,[14] high triglyceride (2.0–4.5 mmol/L [~ 175–400 mg/dL]) and low LDL-C levels, and in nonfasting samples.[15] A study of NHANES, Johns Hopkins, and Mayo Clinic data found that approximately 20% of individuals with LDL-C less than 70 mg/dL (1.8 mmol/L) by the Friedewald equation actually had values greater than or equal to 70 mg/dL (1.8 mmol/L) when compared with the Martin/Hopkins method, reinforcing that the Friedewald formula can lead to underestimation of LDL-C levels, resulting in undertreatment in high-risk patients.[15] In light of the advantages of the Martin/Hopkins method, the clinical laboratory at Johns Hopkins and Quest Diagnostics, among other laboratories, have adopted the Martin/Hopkins method.

CURRENT EVIDENCE: LOW-DENSITY LIPOPROTEIN CHOLESTEROL IN PRIMARY PREVENTION

The risk of cardiovascular disease due to LDL-C is cumulative throughout one's life; thus, primary prevention strategies designed to lower LDL-C should be initiated early in at-risk population to minimize the cumulative lifetime exposure to atherogenic lipoproteins. The goal should not be necessarily to prevent the development of atherosclerosis but rather to slow the rate of progression and delay the development of advanced atherosclerotic plaques that can cause clinical ASCVD.[16]

The American College of Cardiology/American Heart Association (ACC/AHA) guidelines recommend a multifaceted approach to primary prevention through personalized approaches (**Fig. 1**).[15] The guidelines recommend high-intensity statin therapy for adults with severe hypercholesterolemia defined as an LDL-C level greater than or equal to 190 mg/dL in adults between the age of 20 and 75 years. If LDL-C remains elevated despite maximal tolerated statin therapy, ezetimibe or a PCSK9 inhibitor could be considered depending on the level of ASCVD present. The guidelines also recommend statin therapy in patients with diabetes, individuals with 10-year risk greater than or equal to 20%, and selected individuals with 10-year risk of 5% to 19% based on risk enhancing factors and coronary artery calcium.

The guideline recommendations are based on robust evidence.[17] The JUPITER trial studied rosuvastatin in 17,802 individuals with LDL-C less than 130 mg/dL and high-sensitivity C-reactive protein greater than or equal to 2 mg/dL. Rosuvastatin reduced LDL cholesterol levels by roughly 50% from a median 108 mg/dL (2.8 mmol/L) to 55 mg/dL (1.4 mmol/L). The study was terminated early after 1.9 years due to a 44% reduction in all vascular events.[18] The 5-year number needed to treat was 25 among healthy men older than 50 years and 32 among healthy women older than 60 years. In a prospective analysis of JUPITER, participants receiving rosuvastatin who had a baseline LDL-C level less than 70 mg/dL had a 55% reduction in vascular events.[19] In the Collaborative Atorvastatin Diabetes Study, low-intensity atorvastatin reduced cardiovascular disease events including strokes despite the LDL-C level.[20]

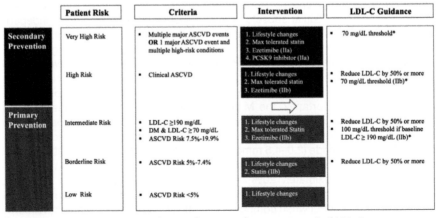

Fig. 1. The ACC/AHA recommendations for treatment target goal of LDL-C.

Multiple studies have evaluated individuals with PCSK9 loss-of-function and familial hypolipidemias.[21] Patients with PCSK9 mutations seem to be healthy and with a significant reduction in coronary events as compared with controls and cardiovascular events are less based on patients' LDL-C levels.[22] The effect may be due to a lifelong low level of LDL-C rather than oscillations, which leads to improved atheroprotection.[23] By way of extrapolation, lowering LDL-C whether by using PCSK9 inhibitors or other lipid-lowering agents earlier in life seems to be a promising primary cardiovascular prevention strategy and perhaps should be incorporated into practice in at-risk individuals.

CURRENT EVIDENCE: LOW-DENSITY LIPOPROTEIN CHOLESTEROL REDUCTION IN SECONDARY PREVENTION

In the 2018 AHA/ACC cholesterol guideline, ASCVD encompasses acute coronary syndrome (ACS), history of myocardial infarction (MI), stable or unstable angina, arterial revascularization, stroke, transient ischemic attack, or peripheral arterial disease (PAD), including aortic aneurysm.[24] The estimated direct and indirect cost of ASCVD in the United States amounts to roughly $219.6 billion per year, and although the incidence of MI and prevalence of coronary artery disease (CAD) have declined significantly as a result of increased efforts at primary and secondary prevention, the prevalence of CAD in the United States remains high (7.2% of adults) with noted discrepancies between ethnicities,[25] and individuals who have had ACS remain at high risk for recurrent ischemic cardiovascular events.[26,27] Similarly, the burden of PAD and stroke remain high, with a lifetime PAD risk of 19%, 22%, and 30% in white, Hispanic, and black individuals, respectively, and roughly 795,000 individuals experience new or recurrent stroke each year, accounting for 1 of every 19 deaths.[25]

The AHA/ACC[25] and European Society of Cardiology/European Atherosclerosis Society (ESC/EAC)[28] guidelines published in 2018 and 2019, respectively, diverge, to some extent, with respect to secondary prevention with the ESC/EAC guidelines being more aggressive (see **Fig. 1**; **Fig. 2**). In the AHA/ACC guidelines, the goal is to reduce LDL-C by greater than or equal to 50% with maximally tolerated statin therapy in individuals with clinical ASCVD. In individuals at very high risk (multiple major ASCVD events or 1 major ASCVD event and multiple high-risk conditions) and LDL-C greater than or equal to 70 mg/dL (1.8 mmol/L) or non–HDL-C greater than or equal to 100 mg/dL (2.6 mmol/L), addition of nonstatin therapies, namely ezetimibe and PCSK9 inhibitors, can be considered.

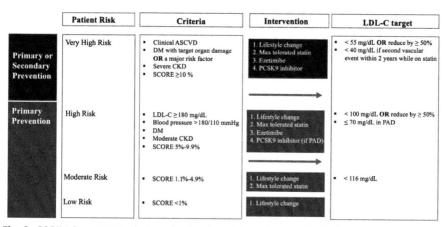

Fig. 2. ESC/EAC recommendations for treatment target goal of LDL-C.

The ESC/EAC categorizes all individuals with ASCVD as "very high risk" (see **Fig. 2**). This categorization extends to individuals without a history of clinical ASCVD but with imaging evidence of ASCVD, including significant plaque on coronary angiography or cardiac computed tomography angiography (multivessel coronary disease with 2 major epicardial arteries having > 50% stenosis) or on carotid ultrasound. For these very-high-risk individuals, LDL-C should be reduced by greater than or equal to 50% from baseline to a goal level of less than 55 mg/dL (<1.4 mmol/L). For those very high-risk individuals who experience a second vascular event within 2 years while on maximally tolerated statin therapy, an LDL-C goal of less than 40 mg/dL (<1.0 mmol/L) should be considered. The ESC/EAC further stated, "the goal should be to reduce LDL-C to as low a level as possible to reduce atherosclerotic risk."

The ESC recommendations echo a slew of recent data showing favorable outcomes with previously unseen reductions in LDL-C in secondary prevention patients (**Table 2**). In the IMPROVE-IT[29] trial, ezetimibe added to statin reduced LDL-C levels from a mean 69.5 mg/dL (1.8 mmol/L) to 53.7 mg/dL (1.4 mmol/L) over 6 years in 18,144 post-ACS patients with an associated decrease in the relative risk of major vascular events by 7.5% with a hazard ratio for clinical benefit per millimole of LDL cholesterol reduction of 0.80. In FOURIER,[30] the PCSK9 inhibitor evolocumab reduced LDL-C from a median 92 mg/dL to 30 mg/dL (0.78 mmol/L) in 27,564 patients with stable ASCVD (either prior myocardial infarction, prior stroke, or symptomatic peripheral artery disease) over a median of 2.2 years, leading to a 15% reduction in the risk of cardiovascular death, myocardial infarction, stroke, hospitalization for unstable angina, or coronary revascularization. In ODYSSEY-OUTCOMES,[31] the PCSK9 inhibitor alirocumab reduced LDL-C from a mean 92 mg/dL to 38 mg/dL (0.98 mmol/L), 42 mg/dL (1.1 mmol/L), and 53 mg/dL (1.4 mmol/L) at 4 months, 12 months, and 48 months, respectively, over a median of 2.8 years in 18,924 patients with ACS 1 to 12 months prior, resulting in a 15% reduction in death from coronary disease, nonfatal myocardial infarction, fatal or nonfatal ischemic stroke, or unstable angina requiring hospitalization. REVEAL[32] studied the cholesteryl ester transfer protein (CETP) inhibitor anacetrapib in 30,449 patients already on a statin with stable ASCVD over a median 4.1 years and showed a reduction in LDL-C from a median 64 mg/dL (1.6 mmol/L) to 38 mg/dL (1.0 mmol/L) with a 9% reduction in the primary outcome of first major coronary event, a composite of coronary death, MI, or coronary revascularization.

A subsequent meta-analysis of IMPROVE-IT, FOURIER, and REVEAL found consistent clinical benefit from further LDL-C lowering in patient populations starting as low as a median of 63 mg/dL (1.6 mg/dL) and achieving levels as low as a median of 21 mg/dL (0.5 mmol/L).[34] The results were similar for statins, ezetimibe, PCSK9 inhibition, and CETP inhibition, despite these drugs having different effects on other risk markers such as HDL, lipoprotein(a), and high-sensitivity C-reactive protein, reinforcing the notion that the reduction in LDL-C (or more broadly, atherogenic apolipoprotein B containing particles) is the primary driver of clinical benefit. Similarly, in a meta-analysis of 19 trials (15 of statins, 3 of PCSK9 inhibitors, and 1 of ezetimibe) with 152,507 patients, each 1.0 mmol/L (~40 mg/dL) reduction in LDL-C was associated with 19% relative decrease in major vascular events over a mean follow-up of 3.95 years.[35]

CURRENT EVIDENCE: LOW-DENSITY LIPOPROTEIN CHOLESTEROL IN CEREBROVASCULAR ACCIDENT

Meta-analyses and randomized controlled trials have demonstrated the benefits of statins in preventing stroke and recurrent stroke in high-risk patients,[36,37] and, similar

Table 2
Recent secondary prevention studies

Trial	Patients	Intervention	Timeframe	Starting LDL-C (mg/dL)	On-treatment LDL-C (mg/dL)	Results
IMPROVE-IT	18,144	Ezetimibe + statin	6 y	69.5 (mean)	53.7	7.5% decrease major vascular events; HR 0.80 of clinical benefit/mmol LDL-C reduction
FOURIER	27,564	Evolocumab + statin	2.2 y	92.0 (median)	30.0	15% reduction in CV death, MI, stoke, hospitalization for unstable angina, or coronary revascularization
EVOPACS	308	Evolocumab + atorvastatin post ACS	8 wk	139.7 (mean)	30.0	Not powered for cardiovascular outcomes
ODYSSEY-OUTCOMES	18,924	Alirocumab + statin	48 mo	92.0 (mean)	53.0	15% reduction in death from CAD, MI, ischemic stroke, or unstable angina requiring hospitalization
SPIRE 1[33]	4556	Bococizumab ± statin	52 wk	94 (mean)	51.8	No MACE benefits
SPIRE 2[33]	5511	Bococizumab ± statin	52 wk	134 (mean)	79.6	HR 0.79 for MACE when LDL-C ≥ 100 mg/dL at baseline
REVEAL	30,449	Anacetrapib + statin	4.1 y	64.0 (mean)	38.0	9% decrease in first major coronary event, composite of coronary death, MI, or coronary revascularization

Abbreviation: HR, hazard ratio.

to CAD, lowering LDL-C to very low levels reduces stroke risk. A recent study of patients with prior ischemic stroke showed patients who had a target LDL-C less than 70 mg/dL had a lower risk of subsequent cardiovascular events than those who had a target range of 90 to 110 mg/dL over 5 years.[38] Meta-regression analysis has shown that each 1 mmol/L decrease in the achieved LDL-C level down to 30.1 mg/dL (0.78 mmol/L) is associated with a 23.5% reduction in stroke risk.[39] In IMPROVE-IT, ezetimibe reduced the frequency of stroke of any cause (hazard ratio [HR] 0.83) and ischemic stroke (HR 0.76) with a particularly large effect seen in patients with a prior stroke (absolute risk reduction 8.6% for stroke of any etiology) without increasing risk of hemorrhagic stroke.[40] Sub-analysis of ODYSSEY-OUTCOMES showed alirocumab reduced the risk of any stroke (HR 0.72) and ischemic stroke (HR 0.73) without increasing hemorrhagic stroke in both patients with and without prior stroke.[41] Furthermore, analysis of FOURIER showed that evolocumab significantly reduced all stroke (HR 0.79) and ischemic stroke (HR 0.75), again with no difference in hemorrhagic stroke.[42]

CURRENT EVIDENCE: LOW-DENSITY LIPOPROTEIN IN PERIPHERAL ARTERIAL DISEASE

LDL-C is a widely accepted causal factor of PAD, which affects 8 to 12 million individuals in the United States and leads to 148,000 major amputations annually.[43,44] Patients with PAD have a heightened risk for having major adverse limb events (MALE), including severe limb ischemia requiring revascularization or amputation, as well as major adverse cardiovascular events (MACE). Despite robust evidence on the benefits of lipid-lowering therapies in reducing the risk for MALE and MACE in PAD, cardioprotective therapies are often underused, with one study showing, relative to CAD alone, patients with PAD alone are less likely to be prescribed antiplatelet drugs, statins, or angiotensin-converting enzyme inhibitors within 18 months of diagnosis.[45]

Statins are first-line therapy for PAD.[46] In the Heart Protection Study, administration of 40 mg simvastatin daily was shown to decrease the rate of first major vascular events by one-quarter and of peripheral vascular events by one-sixth.[46] Similarly, patients with PAD on statins in the REACH (Reduction of Atherothrombosis for Continued Health) registry saw an 18% decrease in the incidence of adverse limb outcomes.[47] Importantly, there was a dose-dependent effect of statins in eliciting significant reduction in limb loss and mortality in PAD.[48]

These findings suggest that statin therapy favorably affects both cardiovascular and limb prognosis in patients with PAD. And the lower the LDL-C levels are in patients with PAD, significantly lower is the risk for adverse cardiovascular and limb outcomes, resulting in very low number needed to treat. In FOURIER, patients with symptomatic PAD had significantly reduced major adverse cardiovascular and limb events.[49] These benefits extended to very low LDL-C values (10 mg/dL) without adverse effects, suggesting that intensive LDL-C lowering is beneficial with symptomatic PAD, including those without concomitant coronary or cerebrovascular disease.

DISCUSSION

LDL-C is increasingly becoming viewed as the garbage product of lipid metabolism. One's total atherosclerotic plaque burden is approximately proportional to his or her cumulative exposure to LDL-C and other apoB-containing lipoproteins. Thus, decreasing the cumulative exposure to these agents has the potential to substantially reduce the number of particles that become retained in the arterial wall and, subsequently, the risk of developing clinical ASCVD. The greater the LDL-C clearance, the better.

Brown and Goldstein suggested that physiologic LDL-C for humans may be in the range of 25 to 60 mg/dL.[50] Levels in that range are present at birth and in adulthood in hunter-gatherer populations with a subsequent very low prevalence of ASCVD.[51,52] Recent arguments posit an LDL-C level of 80 mg/dL may be another possible threshold to achieve ideal cardiovascular health and that, on average, the progression of atherosclerotic plaques stops when LDL-C levels are reduced to less than approximately 70 mg/dL.[16] However, emerging evidence suggests there is no lower limit less than which reducing LDL-C does not show cardiovascular benefit in high-risk patients. FOURIER did not show a cardiovascular benefit plateau, even for LDL-C levels as low as 10 mg/dL, and post hoc spline analysis[53] of ODYSSEY-OUTCOMES showed a decline in all-cause mortality with LDL-C levels down to 30 mg/dL. Although subsequent propensity-score matching analysis[53] of ODYSSEY OUTCOMES showed that those in the alirocumab arm who achieved LDL-C levels less than 25 mg/dL did not derive further reduction in the risk of MACE and all-cause death compared with those who achieved LDL-C levels of 25 to 50 mg/dL, this result is difficult to interpret, given the dynamic changes in lipid therapy and LDL-C introduced by the trial design.

And although there have been concerns regarding increased risk of neurocognitive defects, hemorrhagic stroke, and new-onset diabetes as a sequela of very low LDL-C levels, analyses of PCSK9 trials showed no difference in adverse effects in the experimental and control arms, indicating low LDL-C levels are likely safe.[34,54–58] This notion is further supported by studies showing no increased risk of adverse effects of very low LDL-C levels in individuals with PCSK9 mutations[59] and those undergoing LDL apheresis.[60]

FUTURE DIRECTIONS

There is a continued need for more data on the long-term safety and efficacy of LDL-C lowering therapies. The longest timeline followed was 6 years in IMPROVE-IT. Two long-term extension studies of FOURIER following approximately 6600 patients (NCT03080935 and NCT02867813) are planned to last 5 years and should provide longer-term insights.

SUMMARY

With newer lipid-lowering agents, clinicians now have the armamentarium to robustly and safely lower LDL-C levels and, subsequently, cardiovascular risk. It is important to recognize that atherosclerosis is a chronic, progressive disease that begins early in life and slowly progresses over time before manifesting clinically. With respect to the question of what is the optimal LDL-C, it is not just about how low, but how long, recognizing the importance of cumulative exposure to LDL-C. In general, lower is better and earlier is better. How low to go depends on the patient before you.

CLINICS CARE POINTS

- LDL-C is a well-established, causal factor for ASCVD.
- Long-term exposure to lower LDL-C levels is associated with a lower risk of cardiovascular events compared with shorter-term exposure to lower LDL-C.
- The Friedewald equation is increasingly inaccurate at high triglyceride and low LDL-C levels.

- The Martin/Hopkins method has been validated in patients treated with PCSK9 inhibitors, with diabetes, with familial combined hyperlipidemia, at high triglyceride and low LDL-C levels, and in nonfasting samples.
- Reducing LDL-C with statins in at-risk patients (LDL-C ≥ 190 mg/dL, individuals with diabetes, individuals with 10-year ASCVD risk ≥ 20%, and selected individuals with 10-year risk of 5%–19%) reduces incidence of first ASCVD events.
- Intensively reducing LDL-C with statins, ezetimibe, and PCSK9 inhibitors in patients with clinical ASCVD reduces incidence of recurrent ASCVD events, at least over 5 years.
- Patients achieving very low LDL-C levels see no difference in adverse effects compared with patients with normal LDL-C levels.

DISCLOSURE

A. Gagel, F. Zghyer, and C. Samuel have nothing to disclose. S.S. Martin has research support from the American Heart Association (20SFRN35380046 and COVID19–811000), PCORI (ME-2019C1-15328), National Institutes of Health (P01 HL108800), the Aetna Foundation, the David and June Trone Family Foundation, the Pollin Digital Innovation Fund, the PJ Schafer Cardiovascular Research Fund, Sandra and Larry Small, CASCADE FH, Apple, Google, and Amgen. He has served as a consultant to Akcea, Amgen, AstraZeneca, Esperion, Kaneka, Novo Nordisk, Quest Diagnostics, Regeneron, REGENXBIO, Sanofi, and 89bio. He is a co-inventor on a system to estimate LDL cholesterol levels, patent application pending.

REFERENCES

1. Ference BA, Ginsberg HN, Graham I, et al. Low-density lipoproteins cause atherosclerotic cardiovascular disease. 1. Evidence from genetic, epidemiologic, and clinical studies. A consensus statement fromthe European Atherosclerosis Society Consensus Panel. Eur Heart J 2017;38(32):2459–72.
2. Baigent C, Blackwell L, Emberson J et al. Cholesterol Treatment Trialists' (CTT) Collaboration Efficacy and safety of more intensive lowering of LDL cholesterol: a meta-analysis of data from 170,000 participants in 26 randomised trials. Lancet (London, England). 2010;376(9753):1670–1681. doi:
3. Navarese EP, Robinson JG, Kowalewski M, et al. Association between baseline LDL-C level and total and cardiovascular mortality after LDL-C lowering a systematic review and meta-analysis. JAMA - J Am Med Assoc 2018;319(15):1566–79.
4. Silverman MG, Ference BA, Im K, et al. Association between lowering LDL-C and cardiovascular risk reduction among different therapeutic interventions: A systematic review and meta-analysis. JAMA - J Am Med Assoc 2016;316(12):1289–97.
5. Wang N, Fulcher J, Abeysuriya N, et al. Intensive LDL cholesterol-lowering treatment beyond current recommendations for the prevention of major vascular events: a systematic review and meta-analysis of randomised trials including 327 037 participants. Lancet Diabetes Endocrinol 2020;8(1):36–49.
6. Michos ED, McEvoy JW, Blumenthal RS. Lipid Management for the Prevention of Atherosclerotic Cardiovascular Disease. N Engl J Med 2019;381(16):1557–67.
7. Brownstein AJ, Martin SS. More accurate LDL-C calculation: Externally validated, guideline endorsed. Clin Chim Acta 2020;506(March):149–53.

8. Nauck M, Warnick GR, Rifai N. Methods for measurement of LDL-cholesterol: A critical assessment of direct measurement by homogeneous assays versus calculation. Clin Chem 2002;48(2):236–54.

9. Langlois MR, Nordestgaard BG, Langsted A, et al. Quantifying atherogenic lipoproteins for lipid-lowering strategies: Consensus-based recommendations from EAS and EFLM. Clin Chem Lab Med 2020;58(4):496–517.

10. Martin SS, Blaha MJ, Elshazly MB, et al. NIH Public Access Author Manuscript JAMA. Author manuscript; available in PMC 2014 November 10. Published in final edited form as. JAMA 2013;310(19):2061–8. Comparison of a Novel Method vs the Friedewald Equ. JAMA J Am Med Assoc. 2013;310(19):2061-2068. doi: 10.1001/jama.2013.280532.Comparison.

11. Petridou E, Anagnostopoulos K. Validation of the novel Martin method for LDL cholesterol estimation. Clin Chim Acta 2019;496(June):68–75.

12. Martin SS, Giugliano RP, Murphy SA, et al. Comparison of low-density lipoprotein cholesterol assessment by Martin/Hopkins estimation, friedewald estimation, and preparative ultracentrifugation insights from the FOURIER trial. JAMA Cardiol 2018;3(8):749–53. https://doi.org/10.1001/jamacardio.2018.1533.

13. Chaen H, Kinchiku S, Miyata M, et al. Validity of a novel method for estimation of low-density lipoprotein cholesterol levels in diabetic patients. J Atheroscler Thromb 2016;23(12):1355–64.

14. Mehta R, Reyes-Rodríguez E, Yaxmehen Bello-Chavolla O, et al. Performance of LDL-C calculated with Martin's formula compared to the Friedewald equation in familial combined hyperlipidemia. Atherosclerosis 2018;277:204–10.

15. Sathiyakumar V, Park J, Golozar A, et al. Fasting versus nonfasting and low- density lipoprotein cholesterol accuracy. Circulation 2018;137(1):10–9.

16. Ference BA, Graham I, Tokgozoglu L, et al. Impact of Lipids on Cardiovascular Health: JACC Health Promotion Series. J Am Coll Cardiol 2018;72(10):1141–56.

17. Downs JR, Clearfield M, Weis S, et al. Primary prevention of acute coronary events with lovastatin in men and women with average cholesterol levels: Results of AFCAPS/TexCAPS. J Am Med Assoc 1998;279(20):1615–22.

18. Mora S, Ridker PM. Justification for the use of statins in primary prevention: An intervention trial evaluating rosuvastatin (JUPITER) - Can C-reactive protein be used to target statin therapy in primary prevention? Am J Cardiol 2006;97(2 SUPPL. 1):33–41.

19. Ridker PM, Danielson E, Fonseca FA, et al. Reduction in C-reactive protein and LDL cholesterol and cardiovascular event rates after initiation of rosuvastatin: a prospective study of the JUPITER trial. Lancet (London, England) 2009; 373(9670):1175–82.

20. Colhoun HM, Betteridge DJ, Durrington PN. Primary prevention of cardiovascular disease with atorvastatin in type 2 diabetes in the Collaborative Atorvastatin Diabetes Study (CARDS): Multicentre randomised placebo-controlled trial. ACC Curr J Rev 2004;13(11):34.

21. Minicocci I, Santini S, Cantisani V, et al. Clinical characteristics and plasma lipids in subjects with familial combined hypolipidemia: A pooled analysis. J Lipid Res 2013;54(12):3481–90.

22. Hobbs HH. Sequence Variations in. Hear Dis 2011;1264–72.

23. Karagiannis AD, Mehta A, Dhindsa DS, et al. How low is safe? The frontier of very low (<30 mg/dL) LDL cholesterol. Eur Heart J 2021;1–16.

24. Grundy SM, Stone NJ, Bailey AL, et al. 2018 AHA/ACC/AACVPR/AAPA/ABC/ ACPM/ADA/AGS/APhA/ASPC/NLA/PCNA guideline on the management of blood cholesterol: A Report of the American College of Cardiology/American Heart

Association Task Force on Clinical Practice Guidelines. J Am Coll Cardiol 2019; 139. https://doi.org/10.1161/CIR.0000000000000625.

25. Virani SS, Alonso A, Aparicio HJ, et al. Heart disease and stroke statistics—2021 Update: A Report From the American Heart Association.; 2021. doi:10.1161/cir.0000000000000950

26. Jernberg T, Hasvold P, Henriksson M, et al. Cardiovascular risk in post-myocardial infarction patients: nationwide real world data demonstrate the importance of a long-term perspective. Eur Heart J 2015;36(19):1163–70.

27. Roffi M, Patrono C, Collet JP, et al. 2015 ESC Guidelines for the management of acute coronary syndromes in patients presenting without persistent st-segment elevation: Task force for the management of acute coronary syndromes in patients presenting without persistent ST-segment elevation of. Eur Heart J 2016; 37(3):267–315.

28. Mach F, Baigent C, Catapano AL, et al. 2019 ESC/EAS Guidelines for the management of dyslipidaemias: Lipid modification to reduce cardiovascular risk. Eur Heart J 2020;41(1):111–88.

29. Cannon CP, Blazing MA, Giugliano RP, et al. Ezetimibe added to statin therapy after acute coronary syndromes. N Engl J Med 2015;372(25):2387–97.

30. Sabatine MS, Giugliano RP, Keech AC, et al. Evolocumab and clinical outcomes in patients with cardiovascular disease. N Engl J Med 2017;376(18):1713–22.

31. Schwartz GG, Steg PG, Szarek M, et al. Alirocumab and cardiovascular outcomes after acute coronary syndrome. N Engl J Med 2018;379(22):2097–107.

32. Effects of anacetrapib in patients with atherosclerotic vascular disease. N Engl J Med 2017;377(13):1217–27.

33. Ridker PM, Revkin J, Amarenco P, et al. Cardiovascular efficacy and safety of bococizumab in high-risk patients. N Engl J Med 2017;376(16):1527–39.

34. Sabatine MS, Wiviott SD, Im K, et al. Efficacy and safety of further lowering of low-density lipoprotein cholesterol in patients starting with very low levels: A meta-analysis. JAMA Cardiol 2018;3(9):823–8.

35. Koskinas KC, Siontis GCM, Piccolo R, et al. Effect of statins and non-statin LDL-lowering medications on cardiovascular outcomes in secondary prevention: A meta-analysis of randomized trials. Eur Heart J 2018;39(14):1172–80.

36. Wang W, Zhang B. Statins for the prevention of stroke: A meta-analysis of randomized controlled trials. PLoS One 2014;9(3). https://doi.org/10.1371/journal.pone.0092388.

37. Szarek M, Amarenco P, Callahan A, et al. Atorvastatin Reduces First and Subsequent Vascular Events Across Vascular Territories: The SPARCL Trial. J Am Coll Cardiol 2020;75(17):2110–8.

38. Amarenco P, Kim JS, Labreuche J, et al. A comparison of Two LDL Cholesterol Targets after Ischemic Stroke. N Engl J Med 2020;382(1):9–19.

39. Shin J, Chung J-W, Jang H-S, et al. Achieved low-density lipoprotein cholesterol level and stroke risk: A meta-analysis of 23 randomised trials. Eur J Prev Cardiol 2019. https://doi.org/10.1177/2047487319830503. 2047487319830503.

40. Bohula EA, Wiviott SD, Giugliano RP, et al. Prevention of stroke with the addition of ezetimibe to statin therapy in patients with acute coronary syndrome in IMPROVE-IT (Improved Reduction of Outcomes: Vytorin Efficacy International Trial). Circulation 2017;136(25):2440–50.

41. Jukema JW, Zijlstra LE, Bhatt DL, et al. Effect of alirocumab on stroke in ODYSSEY OUTCOMES. Circulation 2019;140(25):2054–62.

42. Giugliano RP, Pedersen TR, Saver JL, et al. Stroke Prevention with the PCSK9 (Proprotein Convertase Subtilisin-Kexin Type 9) Inhibitor Evolocumab Added to Statin in High-Risk Patients with Stable Atherosclerosis. Stroke 2020;9:1546–54.

43. Norgren L, Hiatt WR, Dormandy JA, et al. Inter-society consensus for the management of peripheral arterial disease (TASC II). J Vasc Surg 2007;45(Suppl S):S5–67.

44. Selby M. Peripheral arterial disease. Pract Nurse 2008;36(7):33–7.

45. Subherwal S, Patel MR, Kober L, et al. Missed opportunities: despite improvement in use of cardioprotective medications among patients with lower-extremity peripheral artery disease, underuse remains. Circulation 2012; 126(11):1345–54.

46. Randomized trial of the effects of cholesterol-lowering with simvastatin on peripheral vascular and other major vascular outcomes in 20,536 people with peripheral arterial disease and other high-risk conditions. J Vasc Surg 2007;45(4):644–5.

47. Kumbhani DJ, Steg PG, Cannon CP, et al. Statin therapy and long-term adverse limb outcomes in patients with peripheral artery disease: insights from the REACH registry. Eur Heart J 2014;35(41):2864–72.

48. Arya S, Khakharia A, Binney ZO, et al. Association of statin dose with amputation and survival in patients with peripheral artery disease. Circulation 2018;137(14): 1435–46.

49. Bonaca MP, Nault P, Giugliano RP, et al. Low-Density Lipoprotein Cholesterol Lowering With Evolocumab and Outcomes in Patients With Peripheral Artery Disease: Insights From the FOURIER Trial (Further Cardiovascular Outcomes Research With PCSK9 Inhibition in Subjects With Elevated Risk). Circulation 2018;137(4):338–50.

50. Brown MS, Goldstein JL. A receptor-mediated pathway for cholesterol homeostasis. Science 1986;232(4746):34–47.

51. O'Keefe JHJ, Cordain L, Harris WH, et al. Optimal low-density lipoprotein is 50 to 70 mg/dl: lower is better and physiologically normal. J Am Coll Cardiol 2004; 43(11):2142–6.

52. Parker CRJ, Carr BR, Simpson ER, et al. Decline in the concentration of low-density lipoprotein-cholesterol in human fetal plasma near term. Metabolism 1983;32(9):919–23.

53. Steg PG, Szarek M, Bhatt DL, et al. Effect of Alirocumab on Mortality after Acute Coronary Syndromes: An Analysis of the ODYSSEY OUTCOMES Randomized Clinical Trial. Circulation 2019;140(2):103–12.

54. Gencer B, Marston NA, Im K, et al. Efficacy and safety of lowering LDL cholesterol in older patients: a systematic review and meta-analysis of randomised controlled trials. Lancet (London, England) 2020;396(10263):1637–43.

55. Giugliano RP, Pedersen TR, Park JG, et al. Clinical efficacy and safety of achieving very low LDL-cholesterol concentrations with the PCSK9 inhibitor evolocumab: a prespecified secondary analysis of the FOURIER trial. Lancet 2017; 390(10106):1962–71.

56. Giugliano RP, Keech A, Murphy SA, et al. Clinical Efficacy and Safety of Evolocumab in High-Risk Patients Receiving a Statin: Secondary Analysis of Patients With Low LDL Cholesterol Levels and in Those Already Receiving a Maximal-Potency Statin in a Randomized Clinical Trial. JAMA Cardiol 2017;2(12):1385–91.

57. Guedeney P, Giustino G, Sorrentino S, et al. Efficacy and safety of alirocumab and evolocumab: a systematic review and meta-analysis of randomized controlled trials. Eur Heart J 2019. https://doi.org/10.1093/eurheartj/ehz430.

58. Gencer B, Mach F, Guo J, et al. Cognition after lowering LDL-Cholesterol With Evolocumab. J Am Coll Cardiol 2020;75(18):2283–93.

59. Benn M, Nordestgaard BG, Grande P, et al. PCSK9 R46L, low-density lipoprotein cholesterol levels, and risk of ischemic heart disease: 3 independent studies and meta-analyses. J Am Coll Cardiol 2010;55(25):2833–42.

60. Kolovou G, Hatzigeorgiou G, Mihas C, et al. Changes in lipids and lipoproteins after selective LDL apheresis (7-year experience). Cholesterol 2012;2012. https://doi.org/10.1155/2012/976578.

Triglycerides
How to Manage Patients with Elevated Triglycerides and When to Refer?

Najdat Bazarbashi, MD[a], Michael Miller, MD[b],*

KEYWORDS

- Hypertriglyceridemia • Remnant particles • Cardiovascular disease
- LDL particle size

KEY POINTS

- Prevalence of HTG in the United states (US) is 25.9%, which is similar to its counterpart nations globally. Very high HTG (TG ≥ 500 mg/dL) represents 1.6% of the US population.
- In recent years, evidence has shown that lower levels of (TG<100) decrease the likelihood of CVD, and incremental increases in TG correspond to a higher mortality risk.
- Triglyceride rich lipoproteins (TRLs) are atherogenic particles and contribute to foam cell formation and atherosclerotic progression via incorporation by macrophages into the arterial lumen.
- Management of HTG is achieved by weight loss, physical activity, dietary changes, and FDA approved therapy including IPE, statins, and fibrates. Novel therapies that target ApoC-III and ANGPTL3 provide encouraging results in clinical trial testing.
- Landmark trials such as EVAPORATE and REDUCE-IT demonstrate supportive evidence for the utilization of purified EPA (Icosapent ethyl) to reduce TG levels, decrease plaque volume and offset MACE.

INTRODUCTION

Hypertriglyceridemia (HTG) is among the most frequent dyslipidemias encountered in modern clinical practice. Causes of HTG include rare genetic disorders, and more commonly, metabolic conditions such as insulin resistance, type 2 diabetes mellitus (T2DM), metabolic syndrome, and central obesity.[1] Untreated HTG contributes to elevated cardiovascular disease (CVD) risk, and in recent years, has been linked to detrimental outcomes.[2,3] On hydrolysis of triglyceride-rich lipoproteins (TRLs), (eg, chylomicrons, very low-density lipoproteins [VLDL]), cholesterol-enriched remnants, the by-products of TRLs, play an important role in the promotion of coronary

[a] Department of Medicine, University of Maryland School of Medicine, Baltimore, MD, USA;
[b] Department of Cardiovascular Medicine, University of Maryland School of Medicine, 110 South Paca Street, Baltimore, MD, USA
* Corresponding author.
E-mail address: mmiller@som.umaryland.edu
Twitter: @mmillermd1 (M.M.)

Med Clin N Am 106 (2022) 299–312
https://doi.org/10.1016/j.mcna.2021.11.006
0025-7125/22/Published by Elsevier Inc.

Abbreviations	
ACCORD	Action to Control Cardiovascular Risk in Diabetes
AIM-HIGH	Atherothrombosis Intervention in Metabolic syndrome with low HDL/high triglycerides: Impact on Global Health outcomes
ARIC	Atherosclerosis Risk in Communities Study
CAC	Coronary Artery Calcium
CVD	Cardiovascular Disease
DHA	Docosahexaenoic Acid
EPA	Eicosapentanoic Acid
EVAPORATE	Effect of icosapent ethyl on progression of coronary atherosclerosis in patients with elevated triglycerides on statin therapy
HDL-C	High-density lipoprotein Cholesterol
HPS2-THRIVE	Heart Protection Study 2-Treatment of HDL to Reduce the Incidence of Vascular Events
HTG	Hypertriglycridemia
IPE	Icosapent Ethyl
LDL-C	Low Density Lipoprotien Cholesterol
LOF	Loss of Function
NFkB	Nuclear Factor - kB
OM3FA	Omega-3 Fatty Acids
PROMINENT	Pemafibrate to Reduce Cardiovascular Outcomes by Reducing Triglycerides
REDUCE-IT	Reduction of Cardiovascular Events with Icosapent Ethyl-Intervention Trial.
STRENGTH	STatin Residual Risk Reduction With EpaNova in HiGh CV Risk Patients With Hypertriglyceridemia
T2DM	Type 2 Diabetes Mellitus
TG	Triglycerides
TRL	Trglyceride Rich Lipoproteins
PPARa	Peroxisome Proliferator-Activated Receptor alpha

atherosclerosis and CVD.[4] Major medical societies recognize HTG as a bonafide CVD risk biomarker, and one recent clinical outcomes trial (ie, REDUCE-IT, described later) demonstrated significant reductions in CVD events in high-risk patients with HTG. In this review, the authors aim to elaborate on the evidence supporting atherogenicity of TRLs, current guidelines recommendations for elevated TGs, and emerging treatment strategies for management of HTG.

Prevalence of Hypertriglyceridemia

The prevalence of HTG (commonly defined as 150 mg/dL and higher) varies across different populations globally and is primarily influenced by genetic predisposition and lifestyle (eg, dietary habits and environmental exposures).[5] For example, a study conducted in China identified 13.8% of the representative sample to have "high" TG ($\geq$200 mg/dL),[6] whereas prevalence of HTG was higher when lower cutpoints were used. Examples include Norway, 26.4% with TG greater than 177 mg/dL and Poland, 21.1%; Russia, 29.2%; and Italy, 27.9% with TG greater than or equal to 150 mg/dL.[7-11] Likewise, prevalence rates were similar in the United States 25.9% with TG greater than or equal to 150 mg/dL based on the National Health and Nutrition Examination Survey with many subjects (6.4 million) exhibiting CVD and T2DM.[12,13]

Triglycerides Cutpoint Revisions

Epidemiologic and other prospective studies examined cutpoints of TG that were most contributory to elevated CVD risk in Western populations. In a meta-analysis of 29 studies (262,525 participants; 10,158 coronary heart disease [CHD] cases) the adjusted odds ratio was 1.72 (95% confidence interval, 1.56–1.90) for TG greater than 180 mg/dL (top tertile) compared with TG less than 120 mg/dL (bottom tertile).[14] A higher likelihood of incident CVD was also observed for TG greater than 166 (upper tertile) versus TG less than 103 (lower tertile) (*P* < .001) in the PROCAM study.[15]

Since 1984, various cutpoints have been established to categorize HTG. For instance, the 1993 National Cholesterol Education Program Guidelines classified TG levels as normal TG less than 200 mg/dL, borderline TG 200 to 399 mg/dL, high TG 400 to 999 mg/dL, and very high TG greater than 1000 mg/dL.[16] Over time, however, these cutpoints have been downwardly adjusted to borderline, 150 to 199 mg/dL; mild-to-moderately high, 200 to 499 mg/dL; and very high, greater than 500 mg/dL.[17] Notably, very high HTG (TG ≥ 500 mg/dL) represents only 1.6% of the US population.[18]

Are Optimal Triglycerides Less Than 100 mg/dL?

As described earlier, HTG is associated with increased CVD risk.[17,19] Although prior guidelines have viewed TG less than 150 mg/dL as desirable, several lines of evidence now suggest that a normal fasting TG level may be lower. For example, in the Baltimore Coronary Observational Long-Term Study compared with higher levels, TG less than 100 mg/dL was associated with a 50% lower likelihood of future CVD events over an 18-year follow-up period.[20] Moreover, a 22-year prospective study of 15,350 patients with established CVD found that compared with baseline TG less than100 mg/dL, there was a correspondingly higher mortality risk of 16%, 29%, and 68% associated with TG levels of 150 to 200, 200 to 499, and greater than or equal to 500 mg/dL, respectively.[21] Finally, a recent combined analysis of the Atherosclerosis Risk in Communities Study (ARIC) and Framingham Offspring Study found that among 8068 men and women without a history of CVD, risk of initial events over a 10-year follow-up period increased across a range of TG levels beginning at levels as low as 50 mg/dL.[22] Taken together, optimal TG levels vis-à-vis CVD risk may be considerably less than 100 mg/dL, thereby mirroring the elevated CVD risk observed with LDL cholesterol as levels exceed 100 mg/dL.

Overview of Triglyceride Metabolism

TRLs are macromolecular complexes composed of cholesteryl esters and triglycerides enclosed by a single layer of apolipoproteins, phospholipids, and free cholesterol.[23] Most TRLs consist of chylomicrons, VLDL, VLDL remnants, and intermediate-density lipoproteins. Chylomicrons are the largest of the TRLs and are derived from dietary fat. They consist of numerous apos (A-I, A-II, A-IV, A-V, B-48, C-II, E), with ApoB-48 viewed as an integral component for secretion into the lymphatics before release in the systemic circulation.[24] VLDLs are composed of apolipoprotein B100 (ApoB-100) and TG. They are produced by hepatocytes and secreted into the circulation whereupon lipoprotein lipase (LPL)-mediated hydrolysis results in the release of free fatty acids (FFAs) that are used as an energy source by peripheral muscle or stored in adipose tissue reserves for subsequent utilization.[17,25]

Mechanisms for High Atherosclerotic Cardiovascular Disease Risk with Hypertriglyceridemia

Remnants incorporated in an unregulated manner (in contrast to low-density lipoprotein)

Although TG is not viewed as atherogenic per se, the primary byproduct of TRLs, cholesterol-enriched remnants, contribute directly to foam cell formation and atherosclerotic progression.[4,26] Analogous to LDL, remnant particles enter the arterial intima, where they become selectively bound to the connective tissue matrix.[27] Once entrapped in the subendothelial space, they are scavenged by resident macrophages in an unregulated manner, thereby contributing to foam cell formation, plaque progression, and potentially, plaque rupture.[27] In contrast to LDL, TRL remnants can be taken up directly by arterial macrophages without oxidative modification and, because of their larger size, carry more cholesterol per particle than LDL.[28] On a particle-per-particle basis, remnants are therefore more atherogenic than LDL.

Apolipoprotein CIII–enriched very low-density lipoprotein particles that promote inflammation

Apolipoprotein CIII (ApoCIII) is a 79-amino acid glycoprotein that plays an integral role in TRL metabolism and atherogenic risk.[17,29] Studies have shown that increased ApoCIII levels in plasma promote vascular inflammation, coronary plaque formation, and worsen cardiac outcomes.[29] ApoCIII regulates lipolysis via noncompetitive inhibition of vascular endothelial-bound LPL, yielding a concentrated environment of small remnant particles that may heighten atherogenic risk,[30,31] in part by upregulating smooth muscle proliferation and activating adhesion molecule-1 (VCAM-1) and NF-kB.[32] By contrast, murine knockout studies found ApoCIII deficiency to enhance hepatic VLDL catabolism by removing its inherent inhibitory effect on LPL.[33] Importantly, loss-of-function (LOF) mutations in *APOC3* resulting in reduced TG/TRL levels as initially demonstrated in an Amish cohort translated into reduced CVD risk so that every 1% lowering of TG corresponded to reduced risk by ∼1%.[34,35] Subsequently, a larger multiethnic study of 6395 individuals found that ApoCIII LOF mutations were associated with significantly reduced TG (43.7%), increased HDL (11.1 g/dL), and lower median (coronary arterial calcification) CAC (27.9 U).[36]

Increased low-density lipoprotein particle concentration/small dense low-density lipoprotein

The molecular size and number of LDL and TRL particles influence the process of atherosclerosis.[37] Insulin resistance (IR) promotes adipocyte FFA release driving hepatic VLDL overproduction.[17] Elevated levels of VLDL-TG activate cholesteryl ester transfer protein (CETP), thereby potentiating TG enrichment of LDL and HDL (**Fig. 1**); this is followed by additional TG hydrolysis by hepatic lipase; the result is a conglomerate of small

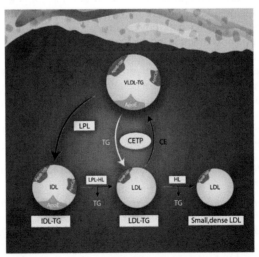

Fig. 1. Metabolic pathway in hypertriglyceridemic state resulting in triglyceride enrichment of LDL. CETP; Cholesteryl Ester Transfer Protein, HL; Hepatic Lipase, IDL; Intermediate Density Lipoprotein, LDL, Low Density Lipoprotein, LPL; Lipoprotein Lipase, TG; triglycerides, VLDL; Very Low Density Lipoprotein.

dense LDL particles possessing low affinity for the LDL-R. With increasing susceptibility to oxidative modification, a proatherogenic milieu ensues with increased uptake and incorporation of cholesterol into the vascular wall.[38]

Triglyceride levels and discordancy between low-density lipoprotein particle size and concentration

Triglyceride levels influence the variability in LDL cholesterol composition. For example, at near-normal TG and LDL cholesterol (LDL-c) (eg, both <100 mg/dL), LDL particles (LDL-p) are predominantly large and normal in composition with minimal discordancy between LDL-p and LDL-c. However, with increasing TG levels, greater exchange of TG for cholesteryl ester molecules occurs within the core of LDL; the extent of these changes is variable and dependent on levels and activity of TG and CETP, respectively. Consequently, the combination of high TG levels and CETP activity not only drives the production of small dense cholesterol-depleted particles but also magnifies the discordancy between LDL-p and LDL-c that in turn may influence atherogenic risk.[39]

Triglyceride enrichment of low-density lipoprotein

As described earlier, certain components of LDL particles influence atherogenicity and play a role in increasing CVD risk including residual elevation in LDL-TG.[40] Previous studies observed a direct association between high levels of LDL-TG and visceral adiposity, angiographically defined coronary disease, T2DM, and vascular inflammation,[41–43] whereas reduced levels of LDL-TG were observed following treatment with the fibrate, gemfibrozil.[44] Most recently, the ARIC study investigated fasting levels of LDL-TG and incident CVD events in a cohort of 9344 individuals affected with the APOE rs7412 variant.[45] The results demonstrated an association between increased levels of LDL-TG and remnant-like particles that correlated with TG levels and CVD risk,[45] although other studies have not confirmed this association.[40,46,47]

Causes of Hypertriglyceridemia

Primary causes

Primary HTG most commonly arises from a group of familial disorders with genetic variants that impair LPL metabolism. Familial combined or mixed hyperlipidemia (type 2B) and dysbetalipoproteinemia (type 3) are among dyslipidemic syndromes presenting with mild-to-moderate HTG (~200–500 mg/dL).[48] Higher TG levels may be observed with LOF mutations in candidate genes affecting TG metabolism (eg, LPL, GP1HBP1, APOA5).[17,49] Some of these rare genetic disorders raise risk of premature CVD.[50,51] As such, screening for familial disorders should be undertaken, especially if responses to TG-lowering therapy are suboptimal (described earlier).

Secondary causes of hypertriglyceridemia including drugs

Secondary HTG most commonly arises from metabolic disorders, sedentary lifestyle, and certain medications (**Box 1**). Obesity and T2DM constitute a large subset of patients with HTG, the latter of which is commonly accompanied by central adiposity, reduced HDL-C, and small dense LDL particles.[17,52] Other causes of HTG include excessive alcohol intake, hypothyroidism, nephrotic syndrome, and drugs such as oral estrogen (tamoxifen), glucocorticoids, antiretrovirals, isotretinoin, second-generation antipsychotics, nonselective β-blockers, and thiazide diuretics.[53,54]

Diagnosis of Hypertriglyceridemia

Although fasting lipid profiles are customary, nonfasting levels have become more popular in recent years,[17,55] especially because they are convenient, reflect real-world metabolic status, and are correlated with fasting levels.[56] Nonfasting samples are being

> **Box 1**
> **Medications that cause hypertriglyceridemia**
>
> Tamoxifen
>
> Oral estrogens
>
> Interferon
>
> Retinoids
>
> Immunosuppressive drugs (cyclosporine, sirolimus)
>
> Raloxifene
>
> Thiazide diuretics
>
> Atypical antipsychotics (fluperlapine, clozapine, olanzapine)
>
> Cyclophosphamide
>
> β-blockers (especially non–beta-1 selective)
>
> Glucocorticoids
>
> L-asparaginase
>
> Bile acid sequestrants
>
> Rosiglitazone
>
> Protease inhibitors

encouraged for general screening, with a repeat fasting lipid profile if the initial screen exceeds 200 mg/dL in the United States[17] or 400 mg/dL in Denmark.[56] The 2018 American College of Cardiology/American Heart Association (ACC/AHA) cholesterol guidelines define HTG as fasting or nonfasting levels between 175 and 499 mg/dL; a level of 175 mg/dL was used instead of 150 mg/dL to adjust for a nonfasting state.[19]

Management of Hypertriglyceridemia

Lifestyle modification

Physical activity. Environmental factors play a significant role in the development and management of HTG. Among these factors, sedentary living is associated with high levels of TG, insulin resistance, and visceral obesity, in large part due to reduced LPL activity.[57] However, increased aerobic physical activity promotes LPL and enhanced lipid oxidation, resulting in advanced hydrolysis and TG utilization by skeletal muscle.[58] Indeed, randomized controlled trials and meta-analyses have shown an inverse relationship between increased aerobic physical activity and TG levels.[17,59–61] Moderate- to high-intensity physical activity, associated with reduced caloric intake, yields an ~20% to 30% reduction in TG levels.[17] Therefore, the recommended physical activity by ACC/AHA (COR 1, LOE B) consists of 150 minutes per week or more of moderate intensity or 75 minutes per week of vigorous intensity.[62]

Dietary Changes

Dietary interventions with careful selection of macronutrient profiles aids in reducing serum TG levels. The type and amount of dietary cholesterol, fat, and alcohol consumed should be reviewed for optimal cardiovascular outcomes. For each kilogram of weight loss achieved, there is an ~8 mg/dL decrease in plasma TG.[62] However, higher baseline TG levels also have the greatest potential for robust TG reductions affected through weight loss in overweight obese patients.[53] Moreover, changes in macronutrient composition (eg, substitution of mono or polyunsaturated fat in place of carbohydrates) may also be effective. For example, a Mediterranean-style diet reduced serum TG by 10% to 15% as compared with individuals on a high-carb diet.[63] In fact, the ACC/AHA recommends a Mediterranean diet inclusive of fruits, vegetables, legumes, nuts, and sandfish to reduce TG and CVD.[62] Further methods of reducing TG levels by dietary changes include the following: the introduction of marine-derived polyunsaturated fatty acids (PUFA) (eicosapentaenoic acid [EPA]/ docosahexaenoic acid [DHA]) to the diet is associated with 5% to 10% reduction in TG, decreasing total carbohydrate intake (1%–2%), and replacement of trans-fatty acids and saturated fatty acids with monounsaturated fatty acids or PUFA (1%).[17,53] In conclusion, a variety of nutritional interventions may be effective and used for long-term improvement in TG levels.[64]

Food and Drug Administration–approved medications: fibrates, niacin, statins, eicosapentaenoic acid

Currently, 4 Food and Drug Administration (FDA)-approved pharmacologic therapies exist for treating HTG. Statins are commonly used as the initial treatment of choice in patients with mild-to-moderate HTG and coexisting T2DM or CVD. On average, statins reduce TG levels 10% to 30%, with greater reductions achieved with high doses of potent statins (eg, atorvastatin 40–80 mg/d, rosuvastatin 20–40 mg/d) as well as high baseline TG levels.[65] In contrast, niacin reduces serum TG by ~20% via inhibition of VLDL synthesis.[66] However, adverse side effects and failure to reduce CVD events has resulted in low utilization of this medication.[67–69] Fibrate therapy is usually well tolerated and reduces serum TG via peroxisome proliferator-activated receptor alpha (PPARα)-mediated activation of LPL, leading to TG reductions ~30% to 50%.[70,71] Although the CVD outcomes trial Action to Control Cardiovascular Risk (ACCORD) failed to demonstrate clinical benefit in patients with T2DM assigned to fenofibrate and simvastatin as compared with simvastatin monotherapy,[72] a prespecified subanalysis revealed a nonsignificant trend in major adverse clinical events favoring fibrate therapy in patients with TG greater than 200 mg/dL and HDL less than 35 mg/dL.[73] A large clinical outcomes trial, the Pemafibrate to Reduce Cardiovascular Outcomes by Reducing Triglycerides (PROMINENT), evaluates the use of the novel fibrate, pemafibrate, in patients with T2DM and/or preexisting CVD to determine whether lowering TG offsets CVD risk in a cohort with HTG and low HDL-C.[74]

Marine-derived omega 3 fatty acids (OM3FA), EPA, and DHA acids reduce TG levels similarly; for each 1 g of OM3 consumed TG levels are reduced 5% to 10%.[17] Icosapent ethyl (IPE), an ultrapurified prescription formulation of EPA, was approved as add-on therapy for patients with TG greater than 500 mg/dL and was tested in a large clinical trial. REDUCE-IT was a phase III double-blind, randomized, placebo-controlled trial evaluating CVD outcomes in 8179 patients with established CVD and high-risk primary prevention patients (aged 50 years and older) with T2DM and at least 1 additional risk factor. Inclusion criteria consisted of fasting TG between 135 and 499 mg/dL and LDL-C between 41 and 100 mg/dL on statin therapy.[75]

Patients were randomized to IPE 4 g/d or a mineral oil placebo over a median follow-up of 4.9 years. The primary endpoint, CVD death, nonfatal stroke, nonfatal myocardial infarction (MI), unstable angina, and coronary revascularization was significantly reduced in IPE-treated patients (hazard ratio 0.75 [0.68–0.83], $P < .001$) with a number needed to treat of 21 patients to prevent one event over the 4.9-year median study period.[75] Interestingly, although there was an ~20% reduction in TG levels in IPE-treated patients compared with controls, this likely contributed to only a small proportion of the benefit observed.[76] Overall, the impressive results of REDUCE-IT expanded IPE's use as a concomitant therapy for the management of patients with TG 150 to 499 mg/dL and CVD or T2DM with at least 1 additional CVD risk factor.[77–79] Consistent with clinical findings of REDUCE-IT was the impact of IPE on progression of coronary low-attenuation plaque volume using multidetector computed tomography in the Effect of Icosapent Ethyl on Progression of Coronary Atherosclerosis in Patients with Elevated Triglycerides on Statin Therapy (EVAPORATE) trial.[80] When compared with placebo, IPE (4 g daily) demonstrated a 17% reduction in low-attenuation plaque (LAP) volume compared with placebo, which demonstrated progression in LAP plaque volume.[80] By contrast, the Effect of High-Dose Omega-3 Fatty Acids versus Corn oil on Major Adverse Cardiovascular Events in Patients at High Cardiovascular Risk (STRENGTH) trial, another outcome trial in patients with high CVD risk with HTG, failed to demonstrate clinical benefit using the combination of EPA and DHA (4 g daily).[81] Most recently, a meta-analysis of 38 randomized controlled trials (n = 149,051) evaluated the effects of DHA and EPA on CVD outcomes and found a higher risk ratio reduction with EPA monotherapy (0.82 [0.68–0.99]) than with EPA + DHA (0.94 [0.89–1.00]) for CVD mortality, nonfatal MI, CHD events, MACE, and revascularization.[82] Basic science studies seem to show divergent properties between EPA and DHA, with EPA exhibiting membrane stabilization, antiinflammatory, antioxidant, and endothelial restorative properties, whereas DHA seems to mitigate this effect.[83] Although more research is warranted to confirm these differences, current data support IPE in patients with preexisting CVD or T2DM with additional CVD risk and HTG.[79,84]

Novel therapies: APOC3 inhibition, ANGPTL3 inhibition, Gemcabene, FGF21
In recent years, there has been an exponential increase in the development of lipid-lowering therapies. Many classes of medications recently approved or are in late-phase clinical trials have focused on treating HTG, including familial disorders. Among the novel therapies are medications that exclusively inhibit apo-CIII including small antisense oligonucleotides (ASOs), monoclonal antibodies, and small interfering RNAs.[30] Volanesorsen, an anti-apoC-III ASO administered subcutaneously, was shown to reduce TG by 77% in patients with familial chylomicronemia syndrome.[85] Despite the significant results, adverse reactions to the medication halted its approval by the FDA. However, second-generation ASO against apo-CIII are underway. Angiopoietin-like protein 3 (ANGPTL3) is a protein involved in the regulation of lipid metabolism mediated through LPL and endothelial lipase.[86] Evinacumab is a monoclonal antibody that inhibits ANGPTL3. Another mechanism involved in ANGPTL3 inhibition therapy is targeted inactivation of messenger RNA (mRNA) via ASO. Both therapies demonstrated a significant reduction in serum TG without major adverse events.[87,88] Gemcabene is a dialkyl ether dicarboxylic acid that reduces hepatic apo-CIII mRNA, which in turn increases the clearance of VLDL, thus making it useful for patients with TG greater than 200 mg/dL.[89] In a phase II study to evaluate the safety and tolerability of gemcabene in subjects with severe hypertriglyceridemia (INDIGO-1) (NCT02944383), gemcabene reduced serum TG by 47% when compared with placebo (27%)[90]; however, it was placed on partial clinical hold due to FDA requirements for murine carcinogenic testing. Fibroblast growth factor 21 (FGF21) is a cytokine involved in cell differentiation, metabolism, and growth via PPARα and PPARζ. Four distinct subtypes of FGF21 have been developed (Pegbelfermin, LY2405319, AMG876/AKR-001, PF-05231023) with various TG-lowering effects.[91] None of the FGF21 therapies have yet to receive FDA approval.

AHA/ACC/ECS/NLA/ADA guidelines recommendation
Management of hypertriglyceridemia according to the 2018 AHA/ACC guidelines is divided into 2 categories. Mild-to-moderate HTG (fasting or nonfasting TG [175–

499 mg/dL] in adults aged 20 years and older is addressed by reducing atherogenic risk factors (eg, T2DM, chronic kidney disease, and medications) in a nonpharmacological manner (COR 1, LOE B).[19] Secondly, in adults aged 40 to 75 years with TG 175 to 499 mg/dL and calculated CVD risk of 7.5% or more, initiation or intensification of statin therapy is recommended after lifestyle, and secondary factors are addressed (COR IIa, LOE B).[19] In contrast, the European College of Cardiology/European Atherosclerosis Society (ECS/EAS) recommends initiation of statin as the drug of choice to reduce CVD risk in high-risk individuals with HTG (>200 mg/dL) (class I, level B).[92] Furthermore, patients who are at high CVD risk with TG (135–499 mg/dL) despite statin treatment should consider IPE 2 g twice a day (class IIa, level B).[92] In other words, the 2018 AHA/ACC guidelines did not recommend additional pharmacologic therapy beyond statins in high-risk patients with elevated TG, whereas the European guidelines supported the addition of IPE.

It is vital to acknowledge that the results of REDUCE-IT trial were released following publication of the 2018 AHA/ACC cholesterol guidelines. Nevertheless, updated statements from the National Lipid Association, ESC/EAS (noted earlier), AHA, and American Diabetes Association now include IPE as adjunctive therapy for reducing CVD risk in high-risk patients with HTG.[78,92–94]

SUMMARY

HTG is a significant risk factor for CVD, even after target LDL-c–lowering goals have been achieved. Identification and treatment of CVD risk factors coexisting with HTG can assist efforts aimed at improving outcomes. In addition to lifestyle measures, management of persistent HTG with statins and IPE may help to offset the excess CVD risk associated with this atherogenic phenotype.

CLINICS CARE POINTS

Hypertriglyceridemia ensues when TG levels rise above 175 mg/dl.

- Optimal TG levels for cardiovascular risk reduction is suggested to be less than 100 mg/dL.
- Nonfasting lipid profile are encouraged for screening of HTG.
- Physical activity and dietary changes are essential to reduce TG levels.
- Statins, IPE, and fibrates are generally recommended as initial pharmacological therapies.
- IPE has a mortality benefit and reduces residual cardiovascular risk in appropriately selected patients.
- Newer therapies (APOC3 inhibition, ANGPTL3 inhibition, Gemcabene, FGF21) are being developed for management of HTG.

DISCLOSURE

Dr M. Miller is a scientific advisor for Amarin, Pfizer, and 89bio. Dr N. Bazarbashi has no disclosures to report.

REFERENCES

1. Rygiel K. Hypertriglyceridemia - common causes, prevention and treatment strategies. Curr Cardiol Rev 2018;14:67–76.
2. Nordestgaard BG, Varbo A. Triglycerides and cardiovascular disease. Lancet 2014;384:626–35.

3. Arca M, Veronesi C, D'Erasmo L, et al. Association of hypertriglyceridemia with all-cause mortality and atherosclerotic cardiovascular events in a low-risk italian population: The TG-REAL retrospective cohort analysis. J Am Heart Assoc 2020;9:e015801.

4. Varbo A, Benn M, Tybjaerg-Hansen A, et al. Elevated remnant cholesterol causes both low-grade inflammation and ischemic heart disease, whereas elevated low-density lipoprotein cholesterol causes ischemic heart disease without inflammation. Circulation 2013;128:1298–309.

5. Sumner AE, Cowie CC. Ethnic differences in the ability of triglyceride levels to identify insulin resistance. Atherosclerosis 2008;196:696–703.

6. Zhang M, Deng Q, Wang L, et al. Prevalence of dyslipidemia and achievement of low-density lipoprotein cholesterol targets in Chinese adults: A nationally representative survey of 163,641 adults. Int J Cardiol 2018;260:196–203.

7. Laufs U, Parhofer KG, Ginsberg HN, et al. Clinical review on triglycerides. Eur Heart J 2020;41:99–109c.

8. Retterstol K, Narverud I, Selmer R, et al. Severe hypertriglyceridemia in Norway: prevalence, clinical and genetic characteristics. Lipids Health Dis 2017;16:115.

9. Zdrojewski T, Solnica B, Cybulska B, et al. Prevalence of lipid abnormalities in Poland. The NATPOL 2011 survey. Kardiol Pol 2016;74:213–23.

10. Karpov Y, Khomitskaya Y. PROMETHEUS: an observational, cross-sectional, retrospective study of hypertriglyceridemia in Russia. Cardiovasc Diabetol 2015;14:115.

11. Giampaoli S, Palmieri L, Donfrancesco C, et al. Cardiovascular health in Italy. Ten-year surveillance of cardiovascular diseases and risk factors: Osservatorio Epidemiologico Cardiovascolare/Health Examination Survey 1998-2012. Eur J Prev Cardiol 2015;22:9–37.

12. Fan W, Philip S, Granowitz C, et al. Prevalence of US Adults with Triglycerides >/= 150 mg/dl: NHANES 2007-2014. Cardiol Ther 2020;9:207–13.

13. Toth PP, Fazio S, Wong ND, et al. Risk of cardiovascular events in patients with hypertriglyceridaemia: A review of real-world evidence. Diabetes Obes Metab 2020;22:279–89.

14. Sarwar N, Danesh J, Eiriksdottir G, et al. Triglycerides and the risk of coronary heart disease: 10,158 incident cases among 262,525 participants in 29 Western prospective studies. Circulation 2007;115:450–8.

15. Assmann G, Schulte H. Relation of high-density lipoprotein cholesterol and triglycerides to incidence of atherosclerotic coronary artery disease (the PROCAM experience). Prospective Cardiovascular Munster study. Am J Cardiol 1992;70:733–7.

16. Summary of the second report of the National Cholesterol Education Program (NCEP) Expert Panel on Detection, Evaluation, and Treatment of High Blood Cholesterol in Adults (Adult Treatment Panel II). JAMA 1993;269:3015–23.

17. Miller M, Stone NJ, Ballantyne C, et al. Triglycerides and cardiovascular disease: a scientific statement from the American Heart Association. Circulation 2011;123:2292–333.

18. Christian JB, Bourgeois N, Snipes R, et al. Prevalence of severe (500 to 2,000 mg/dl) hypertriglyceridemia in United States adults. Am J Cardiol 2011;107:891–7.

19. Grundy SM, Stone NJ, Bailey AL, et al. 2018 AHA/ACC/AACVPR/AAPA/ABC/ACPM/ADA/AGS/APhA/ASPC/NLA/PCNA Guideline on the Management of Blood Cholesterol: A Report of the American College of Cardiology/American Heart Association Task Force on Clinical Practice Guidelines. Circulation 2019;139:e1082–143.

20. Miller M, Seidler A, Moalemi A, et al. Normal triglyceride levels and coronary artery disease events: the Baltimore Coronary Observational Long-Term Study. J Am Coll Cardiol 1998;31:1252–7.

21. Klempfner R, Erez A, Sagit BZ, et al. Elevated Triglyceride Level Is Independently Associated With Increased All-Cause Mortality in Patients With Established Coronary Heart Disease: Twenty-Two-Year Follow-Up of the Bezafibrate Infarction Prevention Study and Registry. Circ Cardiovasc Qual Outcomes 2016;9:100–8.

22. Aberra T, Peterson ED, Pagidipati NJ, et al. The association between triglycerides and incident cardiovascular disease: What is "optimal. J Clin Lipidol 2020;14:438–447 e3.

23. Ginsberg HN. New perspectives on atherogenesis: role of abnormal triglyceride-rich lipoprotein metabolism. Circulation 2002;106:2137–42.

24. Feingold KR, Grunfeld C. Introduction to Lipids and Lipoproteins. In: Feingold KR, Anawalt B, Boyce A, et al., editors. Endotext. South Dartmouth (MA); MDText.com, Inc: 2000.

25. Dallinga-Thie GM, Franssen R, Mooij HL, et al. The metabolism of triglyceride-rich lipoproteins revisited: new players, new insight. Atherosclerosis 2010;211:1–8.

26. Varbo A, Benn M, Tybjaerg-Hansen A, et al. Remnant cholesterol as a causal risk factor for ischemic heart disease. J Am Coll Cardiol 2013;61:427–36.

27. Nordestgaard BG. Triglyceride-Rich Lipoproteins and Atherosclerotic Cardiovascular Disease: New Insights From Epidemiology, Genetics, and Biology. Circ Res 2016;118:547–63.

28. Nakajima K, Nakano T, Tanaka A. The oxidative modification hypothesis of atherosclerosis: the comparison of atherogenic effects on oxidized LDL and remnant lipoproteins in plasma. Clin Chim Acta 2006;367:36–47.

29. Ooi EM, Barrett PH, Chan DC, et al. understanding an emerging cardiovascular risk factor. Clin Sci (Lond) 2008;114:611–24.

30. Taskinen MR, Packard CJ, Boren J. Emerging Evidence that ApoC-III Inhibitors Provide Novel Options to Reduce the Residual CVD. Curr Atheroscler Rep 2019;21:27.

31. Wang CS, McConathy WJ, Kloer HU, et al. Modulation of lipoprotein lipase activity by apolipoproteins. Effect of apolipoprotein C-III. J Clin Invest 1985;75:384–90.

32. Libby P. Triglycerides on the rise: should we swap seats on the seesaw? Eur Heart J 2015;36:774–6.

33. Yan H, Niimi M, Matsuhisa F, et al. Apolipoprotein CIII Deficiency Protects Against Atherosclerosis in Knockout Rabbits. Arterioscler Thromb Vasc Biol 2020;40:2095–107.

34. Crosby J, Peloso GM, Auer PL, et al, Tg, Hdl Working Group of the Exome Sequencing Project NHL. Loss-of-function mutations in APOC3, triglycerides, and coronary disease. N Engl J Med 2014;371:22–31.

35. Pollin TI, Damcott CM, Shen H, et al. A null mutation in human APOC3 confers a favorable plasma lipid profile and apparent cardioprotection. Science 2008;322:1702–5.

36. Natarajan P, Kohli P, Baber U, et al. Association of APOC3 Loss-of-Function Mutations With Plasma Lipids and Subclinical Atherosclerosis: The Multi-Ethnic BioImage Study. J Am Coll Cardiol 2015;66:2053–5.

37. Austin MA, King MC, Vranizan KM, et al. Atherogenic lipoprotein phenotype. A proposed genetic marker for coronary heart disease risk. Circulation 1990;82:495–506.

38. Chait A, Brazg RL, Tribble DL, et al. Susceptibility of small, dense, low-density lipoproteins to oxidative modification in subjects with the atherogenic lipoprotein phenotype, pattern B. Am J Med 1993;94:350–6.

39. Otvos JD, Jeyarajah EJ, Cromwell WC. Measurement issues related to lipoprotein heterogeneity. Am J Cardiol 2002;90:22i–9i.

40. Miller M. Low-Density Lipoprotein Triglycerides: Widening the Atherogenic Landscape in CVD Risk Assessment. J Am Coll Cardiol 2018;72:170–2.

41. Marz W, Scharnagl H, Winkler K, et al. Low-density lipoprotein triglycerides associated with low-grade systemic inflammation, adhesion molecules, and angiographic coronary artery disease: the Ludwigshafen Risk and Cardiovascular Health study. Circulation 2004;110:3068–74.

42. Downing DT. Lipid and protein structures in the permeability barrier of mammalian epidermis. J Lipid Res 1992;33:301–13.

43. Tilly-Kiesi M, Syvanne M, Kuusi T, et al. Abnormalities of low density lipoproteins in normolipidemic type II diabetic and nondiabetic patients with coronary artery disease. J Lipid Res 1992;33:333–42.

44. Olsson AG, Rossner S, Walldius G, et al. Effect of gemfibrozil on lipoprotein concentrations in different types of hyperlipoproteinaemia. Proc R Soc Med 1976;69(Suppl 2):28–31.

45. Saeed A, Feofanova EV, Yu B, et al. Remnant-Like Particle Cholesterol, Low-Density Lipoprotein Triglycerides, and Incident Cardiovascular Disease. J Am Coll Cardiol 2018;72:156–69.

46. Albers JJ, Slee A, Fleg JL, et al. Relationship of baseline HDL subclasses, small dense LDL and LDL triglyceride to cardiovascular events in the AIM-HIGH clinical trial. Atherosclerosis 2016;251:454–9.

47. Varga TV, Kurbasic A, Aine M, et al. Novel genetic loci associated with long-term deterioration in blood lipid concentrations and coronary artery disease in European adults. Int J Epidemiol 2017;46:1211–22.

48. Schaefer JR. Unraveling hyperlipidemia type III (dysbetalipoproteinemia), slowly. Eur J Hum Genet 2009;17:541–2.

49. Dron JS, Wang J, Cao H, et al. Severe hypertriglyceridemia is primarily polygenic. J Clin Lipidol 2019;13:80–8.

50. Brunzell JD, Schrott HG, Motulsky AG, et al. Myocardial infarction in the familial forms of hypertriglyceridemia. Metabolism 1976;25:313–20.

51. Genest JJ Jr, Martin-Munley SS, McNamara JR, et al. Familial lipoprotein disorders in patients with premature coronary artery disease. Circulation 1992;85:2025–33.

52. Fox CS, Massaro JM, Hoffmann U, et al. Abdominal visceral and subcutaneous adipose tissue compartments: association with metabolic risk factors in the Framingham Heart Study. Circulation 2007;116:39–48.

53. Jacobson TA, Ito MK, Maki KC, et al. National Lipid Association recommendations for patient-centered management of dyslipidemia: part 1 - executive summary. J Clin Lipidol 2014;8:473–88.

54. Hegele RA, Ginsberg HN, Chapman MJ, et al. The polygenic nature of hypertriglyceridaemia: implications for definition, diagnosis, and management. Lancet Diabetes Endocrinol 2014;2:655–66.

55. Langsted A, Nordestgaard BG. Nonfasting lipids, lipoproteins, and apolipoproteins in individuals with and without diabetes: 58 434 individuals from the Copenhagen General Population Study. Clin Chem 2011;57:482–9.

56. Nordestgaard BG, Langsted A, Mora S, et al. Fasting is not routinely required for determination of a lipid profile: clinical and laboratory implications including flagging at desirable concentration cut-points-a joint consensus statement from the European Atherosclerosis Society and European Federation of Clinical Chemistry and Laboratory Medicine. Eur Heart J 2016;37:1944–58.

57. Kraegen EW, Cooney GJ, Ye J, et al. Triglycerides, fatty acids and insulin resistance–hyperinsulinemia. Exp Clin Endocrinol Diabetes 2001;109:S516–26.

58. Martin WH 3rd. Effects of acute and chronic exercise on fat metabolism. Exerc Sport Sci Rev 1996;24:203–31.

59. Mann S, Beedie C, Jimenez A. Differential effects of aerobic exercise, resistance training and combined exercise modalities on cholesterol and the lipid profile: review, synthesis and recommendations. Sports Med 2014;44:211–21.

60. Wang Y, Shen L, Xu D. Aerobic exercise reduces triglycerides by targeting apolipoprotein C3 in patients with coronary heart disease. Clin Cardiol 2019;42:56–61.

61. Crichton GE, Alkerwi A. Physical activity, sedentary behavior time and lipid levels in the Observation of Cardiovascular Risk Factors in Luxembourg study. Lipids Health Dis 2015;14:87.

62. Arnett DK, Blumenthal RS, Albert MA, et al. 2019 ACC/AHA Guideline on the Primary Prevention of Cardiovascular Disease: A Report of the American College of Cardiology/American Heart Association Task Force on Clinical Practice Guidelines. J Am Coll Cardiol 2019;74:e177–232.

63. Kastorini CM, Milionis HJ, Esposito K, et al. The effect of Mediterranean diet on metabolic syndrome and its components: a meta-analysis of 50 studies and 534,906 individuals. J Am Coll Cardiol 2011;57:1299–313.

64. Bays HE, Jones PH, Jacobson TA, et al. Lipids and bariatric procedures part 1 of 2: Scientific statement from the National Lipid Association, American Society for Metabolic and Bariatric Surgery, and Obesity Medicine Association: EXECUTIVE SUMMARY. J Clin Lipidol 2016;10:15–32.

65. Stein EA, Lane M, Laskarzewski P. Comparison of statins in hypertriglyceridemia. Am J Cardiol 1998;81:66B–9B.

66. Kamanna VS, Ganji SH, Kashyap ML. Recent advances in niacin and lipid metabolism. Curr Opin Lipidol 2013;24:239–45.

67. Birjmohun RS, Hutten BA, Kastelein JJ, et al. Efficacy and safety of high-density lipoprotein cholesterol-increasing compounds: a meta-analysis of randomized controlled trials. J Am Coll Cardiol 2005;45:185–97.

68. Investigators A-H, Boden WE, Probstfield JL, et al. Niacin in patients with low HDL cholesterol levels receiving intensive statin therapy. N Engl J Med 2011;365:2255–67.

69. Group HTC. HPS2-THRIVE randomized placebo-controlled trial in 25 673 high-risk patients of ER niacin/laropiprant: trial design, pre-specified muscle and liver outcomes, and reasons for stopping study treatment. Eur Heart J 2013;34:1279–91.

70. Sacks FM, Carey VJ, Fruchart JC. Combination lipid therapy in type 2 diabetes. N Engl J Med 2010;363:692–4.

71. Remick J, Weintraub H, Setton R, et al. Fibrate therapy: an update. Cardiol Rev 2008;16:129–41.

72. Group AS, Ginsberg HN, Elam MB, et al. Effects of combination lipid therapy in type 2 diabetes mellitus. N Engl J Med 2010;362:1563–74.

73. Elam M, Lovato LC, Ginsberg H. Role of fibrates in cardiovascular disease prevention, the ACCORD-Lipid perspective. Curr Opin Lipidol 2011;22:55–61.

74. Pradhan AD, Paynter NP, Everett BM, et al. Rationale and design of the Pemafibrate to Reduce Cardiovascular Outcomes by Reducing Triglycerides in Patients with Diabetes (PROMINENT) study. Am Heart J 2018;206:80–93.

75. Bhatt DL, Steg PG, Miller M, et al. Cardiovascular Risk Reduction with Icosapent Ethyl for Hypertriglyceridemia. N Engl J Med 2019;380:11–22.

76. Miller M. Icosapent ethyl for hypertriglyceridemia: insights from the REDUCE-IT Trial. Future Cardiol 2019;15:391–4.

77. FDA. FDA approves use of drug to reduce risk of cardiovascular events in certain adult patient groups. U.S Food and Drug Administration Website; 2019. Available at: https://www.fda.gov/news-events/press-announcements/fda-approves-use-drug-reduce-risk-cardiovascular-events-certain-adult-patient-groups.

78. Orringer CE, Jacobson TA, Maki KC. National Lipid Association Scientific State-ment on the use of icosapent ethyl in statin-treated patients with elevated triglyc-erides and high or very-high ASCVD risk. J Clin Lipidol 2019;13:860–72.

79. Bazarbashi N, Miller M. Icosapent ethyl: drug profile and evidence of reduced re-sidual cardiovascular risk in patients with statin-managed LDL-C cholesterol. Expert Rev Cardiovasc Ther 2020;18:175–80.

80. Budoff MJ, Bhatt DL, Kinninger A, et al. Effect of icosapent ethyl on progression of coronary atherosclerosis in patients with elevated triglycerides on statin ther-apy: final results of the EVAPORATE trial. Eur Heart J 2020;41:3925–32.

81. Nicholls SJ, Lincoff AM, Garcia M, et al. Effect of High-Dose Omega-3 Fatty Acids vs Corn Oil on Major Adverse Cardiovascular Events in Patients at High Cardio-vascular Risk: The STRENGTH Randomized Clinical Trial. JAMA 2020;324: 2268–80.

82. Khan S, Lone AN, Khan MS, et al. Effect of omega-3 fatty acids on cardiovascular outcomes: A systematic review and meta-analysis. 2021;838.

83. Mason RP, Libby P, Bhatt DL. Emerging Mechanisms of Cardiovascular Protec-tion for the Omega-3 Fatty Acid Eicosapentaenoic Acid. Arterioscler Thromb Vasc Biol 2020;40:1135–47.

84. Bazarbashi N, Miller M. Icosapent Ethyl: Niche Drug or for the Masses? Curr Car-diol Rep 2020;22:104.

85. Witztum JL, Gaudet D, Freedman SD, et al. Volanesorsen and Triglyceride Levels in Familial Chylomicronemia Syndrome. N Engl J Med 2019;381:531–42.

86. Mattijssen F, Kersten S. Regulation of triglyceride metabolism by Angiopoietin-like proteins. Biochim Biophys Acta 2012;1821:782–9.

87. Dewey FE, Gusarova V, Dunbar RL, et al. Genetic and pharmacologic inactivation of ANGPTL3 and cardiovascular disease. N Engl J Med 2017;377:211–21.

88. Graham MJ, Lee RG, Brandt TA, et al. Cardiovascular and metabolic effects of ANGPTL3 antisense oligonucleotides. N Engl J Med 2017;377:222–32.

89. Stein E, Bays H, Koren M, et al. Efficacy and safety of gemcabene as add-on to stable statin therapy in hypercholesterolemic patients. J Clin Lipidol 2016;10: 1212–22.

90. Newswire G. Gemcabene meets primary endpoint in INDIGO-1 study of severe hypertriglyceridemia (SHTG) Patients. Globe Newswire: Online; 2018. Available at: https://www.globenewswire.com/news-release/2018/06/28/1531353/0/en/ Gemcabene-Meets-Primary-Endpoint-in-INDIGO-1-Study-of-Severe-Hypertriglyceridemia-SHTG-Patients.html.

91. Geng L, Lam KSL, Xu A. The therapeutic potential of FGF21 in metabolic dis-eases: from bench to clinic. Nat Rev Endocrinol 2020;16:654–67.

92. Mach F, Baigent C, Catapano AL, et al. 2019 ESC/EAS Guidelines for the man-agement of dyslipidaemias: lipid modification to reduce cardiovascular risk. Eur Heart J 2020;41:111–88.

93. Skulas-Ray AC, Wilson PWF, Harris WS, et al. Omega-3 fatty acids for the man-agement of hypertriglyceridemia: a science advisory from the american heart as-sociation. Circulation 2019;140:e673–91.

94. American Diabetes A. 10. Cardiovascular disease and risk management: stan-dards of medical care in diabetes-2020. Diabetes Care 2020;43:S111–34.

Cardiovascular Genetics
The Role of Genetics in Predicting Risk

Jessica Chowns, CGC*, Lily Hoffman-Andrews, CGC,
Amy Marzolf, CRNP, Nosheen Reza, MD, Anjali Tiku Owens, MD*

KEYWORDS

- Genetic testing • Cardiovascular genetics • Cascade screening
- Inherited cardiovascular disease • Genetic counseling • Precision medicine

KEY POINTS

- Genetic testing is recommended by guidelines for many cardiovascular conditions and is useful for diagnosis, management, and cascade screening.
- Genetic testing for cardiovascular conditions in healthy people with no family history is not widely recommended at this time.
- Appropriate pretest and posttest genetic counseling are crucial because of the complexity of genetic information and its implications for patients and their families.

INTRODUCTION

Most primary care physicians have been or will be asked about genetic testing by their patients, but many do not feel adequately prepared to discuss this topic.[1,2] Some patients may have no personal or family history of a potentially genetic disease but are interested in learning about their genetic risk. In years past, high cost of clinical genetic testing was often a barrier, but with the progress in genetic testing technologies, cost has decreased and genetic testing is increasingly being performed in those with suspected genetic cardiovascular diseases as well as in some healthy people. There is still much to learn about the genetic risk factors that influence cardiovascular disease development, as well as how we might seek to mitigate that risk. In this review, we provide information about genetic testing for cardiovascular diseases and a framework for primary care physicians and their teams to better understand situations in which genetic testing may contribute important information to patient care.

Division of Cardiovascular Medicine, Department of Medicine, Center for Inherited Cardiovascular Disease, Perelman School of Medicine at the University of Pennsylvania, Perelman Center for Advanced Medicine, 3400 Civic Center Boulevard, 11th Floor South Pavilion, Philadelphia, PA 19104, USA
* Corresponding authors.
E-mail addresses: Jessica.chowns@pennmedicine.upenn.edu (J.C.); anjali.owens@pennmedicine.upenn.edu (A.T.O.)

Med Clin N Am 106 (2022) 313–324
https://doi.org/10.1016/j.mcna.2021.11.007
0025-7125/22/Published by Elsevier Inc.

GENETIC TESTING
For Which Types of Cardiovascular Conditions Should Genetic Testing Be Offered?

Many professional societies have published guidelines on genetic evaluation in cardiovascular diseases, and genetic testing is recommended for many cardiovascular phenotypes. The American Heart Association and other professional societies have recognized that cardiogenetic evaluation requires specific expertise and is best performed in the setting of a multidisciplinary specialist clinic.[3] Team members in these clinics include cardiologists, advanced practitioners, and genetic counselors with expertise in cardiovascular genetics among others (**Fig. 1**). Obtaining a detailed three-generation family history is of utmost importance in the genetic evaluation of cardiovascular disease. This information can greatly impact the care of patients and their families more than genetic testing can in some cases.

Cardiovascular genetic testing can be helpful for risk stratification or providing management guidance in some with cardiovascular disease and is also helpful for reproductive planning and aiding in cascade screening of at-risk family members. In most cases, a diagnosis is made based on clinical cardiovascular testing. However, the presence of a causative genetic variant can be part of the diagnostic criteria for certain conditions, including catecholaminergic polymorphic ventricular tachycardia, arrhythmogenic right ventricular cardiomyopathy, Loeys-Dietz syndrome, and Marfan syndrome. For some conditions, genetic test results can aid in risk prediction for clinical events and may impact the choice of medical therapy or timing of certain interventions. There are some conditions, however, like atrial fibrillation, for which genetic testing is not typically recommended. Because the paradigm of genetic testing is probabilistic and not deterministic, negative genetic test results on a proband with disease can almost never rule out a genetic predisposition. The degree to which genetic test results can be helpful as well as the detection rate, or the likelihood of identifying a genetic cause, can also vary greatly by phenotype. We summarize this information for selected cardiovascular phenotypes in **Table 1**.

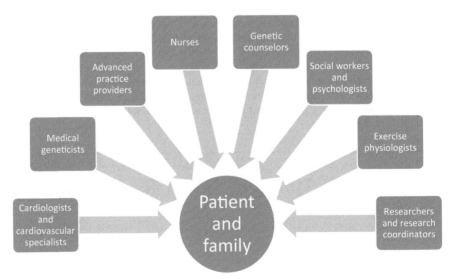

Fig. 1. Members of a multidisciplinary cardiogenetics team.

Table 1
Genetic testing for select cardiovascular phenotypes

Phenotype	Guidelines Supporting Genetic Testing	Yield of Genetic Testing	Potential Impact on Medical Management
Cardiomyopathies HCM DCM ACM	HFSA[20] HRS/EHRA[21]	HCM: 30%–60% DCM: 30%–40% ACM: ~60%	Rare[a]

Arrhythmia
  conditions LQTS
BrS
CPVT
	HRS/EHRA[22]	LQTS: 50%–75%
		BrS (SCN5A):
		  20%–25%
		CPVT: ~50%
			Yes

Sudden cardiac
  death/ventricular
  arrhythmias
	HRS/EHRA[22]
	APHRS/HRS[23]
		15–30%[b]	Yes

FTAAD	ACCF/AHA[24]	10–20%[c]	Yes
Familial hypercholesterolemia	NICE[25] NLA[26]	60%–80%	Yes

Abbreviations: ACCF, American College of Cardiology Foundation; ACM, arrhythmogenic cardiomyopathy (including ARVC/D); AHA, American Heart Association; APHRS, Asia Pacific Heart Rhythm Society; ARVC/D, arrhythmogenic right ventricular cardiomyopathy/dysplasia; BrS, Brugada syndrome; CPVT, catecholaminergic polymorphic ventricular tachycardia; DCM, dilated cardiomyopathy; EHRA, European Heart Rhythm Association; FTAAD, familial aortic aneurysms and dissections; HCM, hypertrophic cardiomyopathy; HFSA, Heart Failure Society of America; HRS, Heart Rhythm Society; NICE, National Institute for Health and Care Excellence; NLA, National Lipid Association; LMNA, lamin A/C (gene); LQTS, long QT syndrome; TTR, transthyretin (gene).
  [a] Exceptions include LMNA, ACM genes and phenocopies of HCM, including TTR cardiac amyloidosis, and Fabry disease.
  [b] In cases of sudden unexplained death (autopsy-negative sudden death).
  [c] Yield is higher in those with Marfan syndrome and other syndromic forms of aortopathy.

Selecting the Appropriate Individual for Genetic Testing

All major guidelines for cardiovascular genetic testing recommend that the proband, or individual selected for the initiation of genetic testing in a family, be an individual affected with the disease. Ideally, this should also be the person in the family who is most severely affected and/or has the earliest age of onset, because this increases the likelihood of finding an informative result (**Fig. 2**).

Genetic testing of unaffected individuals should only be performed for risk stratification when a causative variant has been identified in the family, and testing should be limited to that variant. Genetic testing of unaffected individuals as probands is not currently recommended for cardiovascular conditions, even when an affected family member is not available for testing. Because the yield of genetic testing for cardiovascular conditions is incomplete, negative genetic testing results from an unaffected person when a causative variant has not been identified in the family are uninformative: it is impossible to know, without testing the affected family member, whether the result is a true-negative or if there is a genetic predisposition present that is not identifiable on current testing. These uninformative negative results may, nonetheless, lead to false reassurance or inappropriate management by nonspecialist clinicians. A positive result, on the other hand, rarely changes management compared with screening recommendations guided by family history alone, and it can be difficult to confidently attribute disease in a family to a variant that has not been confirmed in affected individuals. In

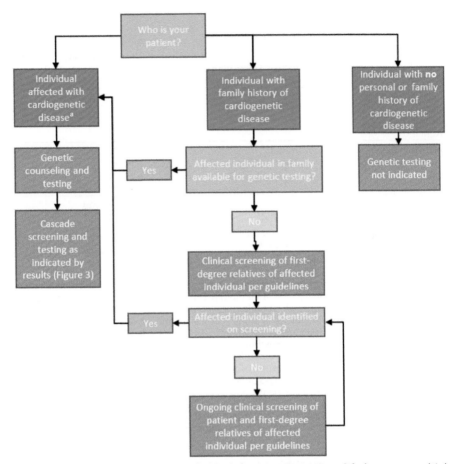

Fig. 2. Choosing the appropriate individual for genetic testing. [a]If there are multiple affected individuals in the family, testing should ideally start with the individual who is most severely affected and/or had the youngest age of onset.

addition, the challenges of uncertain genetic test results, discussed in more detail in later sections, are even greater when testing unaffected individuals and may produce unnecessary anxiety and uncertainty. Genetic testing of unaffected individuals as probands is performed more often in cancer genetics because there are well-defined guidelines for such and genetic test results more often impact medical management. It is possible that this may one day be the case for cardiac conditions as well.

CASCADE SCREENING

Cascade screening is a process whereby family members are evaluated for a disease that runs in their family (**Fig. 3**). Cascade screening can involve either clinical screening or genetic testing, depending on the genetic test results of the proband. When genetic testing is used for this purpose, it is important that there is confidence that the genetic variant identified is actually causing the familial disease phenotype. Most genetic cardiovascular diseases are inherited in an autosomal dominant pattern such that all first-degree family members have a 50% chance of inheriting the genetic predisposition to develop disease regardless of sex. In most cases, a

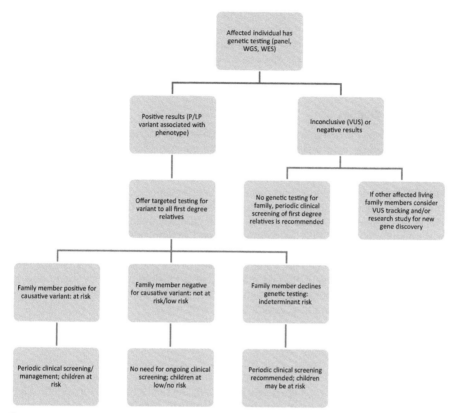

Fig. 3. Cascade screening. LP, likely pathogenic variant; P, pathogenic variant; VUS, variant of uncertain significance; WES, whole-exome sequencing; WGS, whole-genome sequencing.

causative variant was inherited from a parent, and determining which parent allows for further cascade screening of appropriate aunts, uncles, and cousins of the proband. Testing children younger than 18 years of age for pathogenic variants in genes associated with cardiovascular disease can be considered, but special attention should be paid to whether the results will truly impact their management with consideration of the potential positive and negative effects of genetic testing. If families decide that the risks of genetic testing for their children outweigh the benefits, they can defer or forgo genetic testing and continue with periodic clinical screening to see if the disease phenotype emerges.

Owing to regulations imposed by the Health Insurance Portability and Accountability Act of 1996 (HIPAA), providers cannot reach out to family members at risk for disease directly, so the responsibility of informing family members of their risk lies primarily with patients in the vast majority of cases. In many clinics, genetic counselors write letters to help patients communicate this information with their families, but there are often family members who do not pursue cascade screening. As such, there are ongoing efforts to develop other ways of helping patients communicate this information.[4]

Some genetic causes of cardiovascular disease are fully penetrant, meaning that nearly everyone with the causative variant will develop some manifestation of disease, whereas most exhibit reduced penetrance and variable expressivity. For many cardiovascular risk genes and variants within those genes, precise penetrance estimates are still lacking; this can further complicate discussions surrounding cascade screening. Expert consensus groups including ClinGen are trying to better characterize risk of developing disease by gene and/or variant, but it will likely be many years before better risk estimates for most cardiovascular genetic conditions are available.[5]

Reproductive Options

Prenatal testing, including chorionic villus sampling (CVS) and amniocentesis, and preimplantation genetic testing for monogenic disease (PGT-M) were options first used for couples who were both carriers for the same recessive genetic conditions to ensure any children they had were not born with the disease or at risk for disease. In recent years, these technologies have been used in various cardiovascular diseases for which the genetic cause has been successfully identified. CVS and amniocentesis involve taking placental tissue or amniotic fluid samples, respectively, to test a fetus for a genetic condition. PGT-M, formerly termed preimplantation genetic diagnosis (PGD), requires the use of in vitro fertilization (IVF) to create embryos that are then tested for the causative genetic variant to determine if the embryo will be used for conception. Doing IVF with PGT-M may not be a feasible option for many due to high cost, but some insurance companies cover at least part of the cost, and there are clinical trials providing this service at low or no cost.

SELECTING THE APPROPRIATE GENETIC TEST
Panel Testing

Most genetic cardiovascular disorders have multiple possible genetic causes, and therefore assessment of multiple genes is typically the best approach for genetic diagnosis. At present, the most common type of diagnostic genetic testing for cardiovascular conditions is panel testing, in which a set of genes relevant to the patient's phenotype are sequenced. When the phenotype is well defined, a narrow panel is most appropriate; broader panels may be helpful when the phenotype is less well defined, but they also increase the likelihood of uncertain or unrelated findings. The genes included on panels vary between laboratories and change over time, as new gene-disease associations are discovered.

Single-Gene and Single-Variant Testing

Single-gene testing may be appropriate when clinical suspicion is very high for a disorder caused by only one gene (eg, *TTR* in hereditary transthyretin amyloidosis). Single-variant testing, in which the presence or absence of a specific variant within a gene is assessed, is the appropriate test for family members when a causative variant has been identified in the family.

Whole-Exome and Whole-Genome Sequencing

Whole-exome sequencing (WES) and whole-genome sequencing (WGS), in which a patient's protein-coding genes or entire DNA sequence, respectively, are analyzed, are currently of limited utility in adult cardiovascular care settings: they increase diagnostic yield only very modestly compared with panels and create a significantly greater burden of uncertainty.[6,7] However, they are more commonly used, and have more utility, in pediatric settings and/or when syndromic or multisystem disease is present. In addition, WES and WGS are commonly used in research studies and are useful for gene discovery.

Direct-to-Consumer Genetic Testing

Direct-to-consumer (DTC) genetic testing has grown rapidly in recent years. The first wave of DTC genetic tests were offered without the need for a physician's approval, and often include health-related genetic data along with ancestry or other information. A newer model of DTC testing includes physician involvement; tests may be ordered by the patient's own physician or by a physician employed by the DTC company. This type of testing is often referred to as "proactive" testing and is typically marketed to healthy individuals who want to learn more about their genetic predisposition to disease. Tests consist of genetic panels with genes selected for actionability, especially those associated with cardiovascular and cancer risk.[8] Some major academic health care systems have recently made such tests available to their students and staff at no cost to them. Some DTC companies also provide patients access to their raw genetic data, which can be analyzed with the help of third-party services. Despite the perceived benefits of this open information exchange, these third-party analyses have been shown to lead to false-positive results.[9] There are currently no guidelines for how clinicians should approach DTC testing. The clinical utility of DTC tests has not been comprehensively studied, and this represents an emerging need in genetics.[10]

Polygenic Risk Scores

Common cardiovascular diseases, including coronary artery disease, stroke, and atrial fibrillation, are known to have both environmental and familial components but typically do not have mendelian (single-gene) causes. Instead, the hereditary aspect is thought to arise from many common genetic variants, each with a small individual contribution to risk. Genome-wide association studies (GWAS) have been able to identify some of the common genetic variation underlying these conditions. In turn, polygenic risk scores (PRS) are tools that use information gleaned from GWAS to attempt to better risk stratify individuals for these disorders by genotyping them for common genetic variation. Despite growing interest in PRS and evidence suggesting that it can contribute to risk prediction for various common disorders, their clinical utility is limited at this time and there is not yet established guidance for if and how PRS should be used in practice.[11]

POSSIBLE RESULTS FROM GENETIC TESTING

Variant interpretation is one of the more challenging aspects of clinical genetics. There is a great deal of genetic variation between individuals, most of which is benign. Distinguishing pathogenic from benign variation identified on genetic testing relies on multiple lines of evidence including case reports, population prevalence data, and computational and laboratory evidence. Classifying variants is generally the purview of the genetic testing laboratory, but laboratories do not always agree on variant interpretation. In 2015, to help address this issue of discordant variant classifications between laboratories and provide standardized guidance for variant assessment, the American College of Medical Genetics and Genomics (ACMG) and the Association for Molecular Pathology issued updated guidelines for classification of sequence variants providing detailed criteria by which laboratories should classify variants into 5 categories: pathogenic (P), likely pathogenic (LP), variant of uncertain significance (VUS), likely benign (LB), and benign (B). LP and LB variants are defined as having a greater than 90% likelihood of being pathogenic or benign, respectively, whereas a VUS falls in the middle range of 10% to 90%.

P and LP variants can contribute to diagnosis, management, and familial risk stratification, although clinical correlation is important, because P or LP variants may sometimes be incidental findings that are not truly related to the indication for testing. VUS findings mean that evidence is insufficient or conflicting about the pathogenicity of the variant, and the variant cannot confidently be classified as pathogenic or benign. VUS results are very common in cardiovascular genetics and should not be used to guide management or risk stratify family members. B and LB variants are not associated with disease and are typically not reported by clinical laboratories.

Even with the detailed guidance offered by ACMG, variant classification is a complex art, and laboratories still often differ in their interpretation. Efforts to further harmonize and improve variant classification are ongoing. The ClinGen consortium, founded by the National Human Genome Research Institute in 2013, maintains the public ClinVar database wherein laboratories and other groups publicly share their variant classifications and organizes gene- and condition-specific working groups to review evidence for genes and variants.[12] Another important resource for variant classification is population prevalence data on genetic variants; the Genome Aggregation Database (gnomAD) is a public database of variant frequency in thousands of exomes and genomes of individuals unselected for disease, from multiple ethnicities.[13] Although gnomAD has improved variant interpretation in minority populations, there is still greater potential for misdiagnoses based on genetic test results in minority populations.[14]

Clinicians with expertise in cardiovascular genetics often take an active role in variant interpretation by aggregating additional information on variants reported on genetic testing.[15] To further elucidate VUS, clinicians may undertake additional investigations, including tracking VUS in affected family members to determine whether variants segregate with disease.

Variant Reinterpretation

The classification of variants can change over time as new data emerge. Variants may be upgraded or downgraded in their level of pathogenicity, which can have significant impact on management, especially in family members. There has been much debate on who has responsibility to stay abreast of potential changes in variant interpretation. Some have suggested that the responsibility lies with the genetic testing laboratories and others with clinicians. There are no clear guidelines on who maintains this responsibility, when to recontact patients, or how often to perform variant re-interpretation, but most recognize these tasks need to be performed periodically.[16,17] At present, clinical genetic testing laboratories are not routinely reinterpreting genetic variants but will do so when requested by a clinician or genetic counselor.[18] If a variant is identified in numerous individuals at one laboratory and a change in interpretation occurs over time, the laboratories do have procedures in place to disseminate updated reports or contact the ordering provider for every patient with that variant identified at their laboratory. However, if a patient has moved or a clinician is no longer practicing at that location, communicating that variant update can be challenging. In our clinic, our genetic counselors handle much of these responsibilities, which can occupy a significant amount of non-face-to-face clinical time. In clinics with no or limited genetic counselor support, these responsibilities can fall on clinicians themselves or their staff, but in many clinics these tasks may never be performed.

COMMON CONCERNS REGARDING GENETIC TESTING
Discrimination and Privacy

Concerns over discrimination based on genetic information have been raised for decades and continue to be of concern, especially with the increasing availability of genetic testing. There are many state and federal protections in place in the United States, but gaps exist and discrimination may still occur. One such piece of federal protections legislation is the Genetic Information Nondiscrimination Act (GINA), which became law in 2008. GINA protects against employment and health insurance discrimination based on genetic information. Protected genetic information includes family history, participation in genetic research, genetic test results, and the use of genetic counseling and other services.[19] GINA does not protect against life insurance, long-term care insurance, or disability insurance discrimination, and few state laws exist to protect people from discrimination for these types of policies. Consequently, some individuals chose to obtain these types of insurances before undergoing cascade screening. GINA does not apply to all groups; exclusions include people in the military or those who work at a company with less than 15 employees.[19]

In the United States, HIPAA requires that clinicians and clinical genetic testing laboratories keep patients' test results, including genetic test results, confidential in most cases. Although the risk for patient's privacy related to genetic testing performed at a clinical genetic testing laboratory is very low due to HIPAA and its protections, patients may express reluctance to undergo genetic testing due to privacy concerns such as access of genetic information by law enforcement or by previously unknown biological relatives, typically associated with DTC testing.

Cost

The cost of genetic testing is often highest for probands and currently ranges from $250 to a few thousand dollars, depending on the genetic test ordered (highest for WGS and WES, lowest for panels) and insurance coverage. If a pathogenic variant is identified in a proband, testing family members for just that variant can sometimes be done for free or at much lower cost depending on insurance coverage and genetic testing laboratory policy. Cost and access still remain as barriers, but these have improved significantly.

CASE STUDY

A 58-year-old man of European ancestry with a history of idiopathic dilated cardiomyopathy (DCM) presented for consideration of genetic testing. Although he did not report a clear family history of similar concerns (**Fig. 4**), genetic testing for cardiomyopathy risk genes was pursued. Genetic testing identified 2 VUSs, which could not be used to risk stratify his family members, and periodic clinical screening for DCM was recommended for his first-degree relatives. After a few years, we reanalyzed his results and one of the variants was downgraded to likely benign, whereas the other was upgraded to pathogenic. Unfortunately, the patient died due to complications of heart transplantation. His 3 children then presented to clinic for evaluation, and targeted genetic testing for the pathogenic variant identified in their father was offered. All 3 were negative for the pathogenic variant and dismissed from ongoing cardiac surveillance.

Case Study Discussion

VUSs are common in cardiovascular genetics and need to be reevaluated periodically, and genetic testing in appropriate probands yields the most helpful results. If we had not tested the appropriate genetic testing proband (the father) first and offered panel testing to each of his children instead, their results would have been negative or additional VUSs could have been identified. In that scenario, we would not have known that

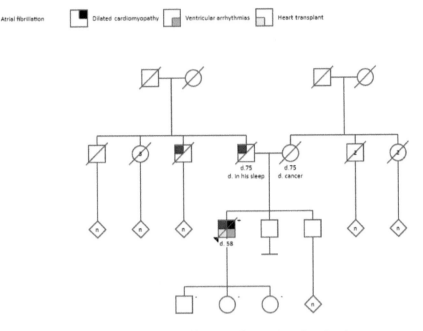

(+) = Positive for causative pathogenic variant; (-) = negative for causative pathogenic variant

Fig. 4. Pedigree. +, Positive for causative pathogenic variant; −, negative for causative pathogenic variant.

they were truly not at risk and they would have been recommended to continue with periodic clinical screening for DCM.

SUMMARY

Genetic testing for selected cardiovascular conditions can be helpful for patients and their families, but it is far from perfect. Understanding the complexities of the genetics of cardiovascular disease and the implications of such can make counseling about genetic risk of cardiovascular disease challenging even for the most-well-trained professionals. Genetic testing is integral to the goal of achieving truly personalized care for our patients, and to do it appropriately requires significant training and multidisciplinary expertise.

CLINICS CARE POINTS

- Genetic testing for selected cardiovascular phenotypes can provide useful clinical information for affected individuals and allow for cascade screening in unaffected relatives.
- Cardiovascular genetic testing in healthy individuals outside of cascade screening is generally not recommended at this time but is available.
- VUSs are common in cardiovascular genetics and should not be used for clinical management or cascade screening.
- Genetic test results need to be periodically reevaluated for potential updates in variant interpretation.

DISCLOSURE

Dr A.T. Owens is a consultant for MyoKardia and Cytokinetics and receives funding from the Winkelman Family Fund for Innovation. Dr N. Reza is supported by the National Center for Advancing Translational Sciences of the National Institutes of Health under award number KL2TR001879. The content is solely the responsibility of the authors and does not necessarily represent the official views of the National Institutes of Health.

REFERENCES

1. Bonter K, Desjardins C, Currier N, et al. Personalised medicine in Canada: a survey of adoption and practice in oncology, cardiology and family medicine. BMJ Open 2011;1(1):e000110.
2. Mainous AG 3rd, Johnson SP, Chirina S, et al. Academic family physicians' perception of genetic testing and integration into practice: a CERA study. Fam Med 2013;45(4):257–62.
3. Ahmad F, McNally Elizabeth M, Ackerman MJ, et al. Establishment of Specialized Clinical Cardiovascular Genetics Programs: Recognizing the Need and Meeting Standards: A Scientific Statement From the American Heart Association. Circ Genomic Precis Med 2019;12(6):e000054.
4. Ingles J, Semsarian C. Making the case for cascade screening among families with inherited heart disease. Heart Rhythm 2020;17(1):113–4.
5. Adaptation and validation of the ACMG/AMP variant classification framework for MYH7-associated inherited cardiomyopathies: recommendations by ClinGen's Inherited Cardiomyopathy Expert Panel - ClinGen | Clinical Genome Resource. Available at: https://www.clinicalgenome.org/docs/adaptation-and-validation-of-the-acmg-amp-variant-classification-framework-for-myh7-associated-inherited-cardiomyopathies/. Accessed April 16, 2021.
6. Minoche AE, Horvat C, Johnson R, et al. Genome sequencing as a first-line genetic test in familial dilated cardiomyopathy. Genet Med 2019;21(3):650–62.
7. Cirino Allison L, Lakdawala Neal K, Barbara M, et al. A Comparison of Whole Genome Sequencing to Multigene Panel Testing in Hypertrophic Cardiomyopathy Patients. Circ Cardiovasc Genet 2017;10(5):e001768.
8. Kalia SS, Adelman K, Bale SJ, et al. Recommendations for reporting of secondary findings in clinical exome and genome sequencing, 2016 update (ACMG SF v2.0): a policy statement of the American College of Medical Genetics and Genomics. Genet Med 2017;19(2):249–55.
9. Tandy-Connor S, Guiltinan J, Krempely K, et al. False-positive results released by direct-to-consumer genetic tests highlight the importance of clinical confirmation testing for appropriate patient care. Genet Med 2018;20(12):1515–21.
10. Myers M, Bloss C. The need for education and clinical best practice guidelines in the era of direct-to-consumer genomic testing. JMIR Med Educ 2020;6(2):e21787.
11. Lewis CM, Vassos E. Polygenic risk scores: from research tools to clinical instruments. Genome Med 2020;12(1):44.
12. Landrum MJ, Lee JM, Benson M, et al. ClinVar: improving access to variant interpretations and supporting evidence. Nucleic Acids Res 2018;46(D1):D1062–7.
13. Karczewski KJ, Francioli LC, Tiao G, et al. The mutational constraint spectrum quantified from variation in 141,456 humans. Nature 2020;581(7809):434–43.
14. Manrai AK, Funke BH, Rehm HL, et al. Genetic Misdiagnoses and the Potential for Health Disparities. N Engl J Med 2016;375(7):655–65.

15. Reuter C, Grove ME, Orland K, et al. Clinical Cardiovascular Genetic Counselors Take a Leading Role in Team-based Variant Classification. J Genet Couns 2018; 27(4):751–60.
16. Stevens YA, Senner GD, Marchant GE. Physicians' duty to recontact and update genetic advice. Pers Med 2017;14(4):367–74.
17. David KL, Best RG, Brenman LM, et al. Patient re-contact after revision of genomic test results: points to consider—a statement of the American College of Medical Genetics and Genomics (ACMG). Genet Med 2019;21(4):769–71.
18. Chisholm C, Daoud H, Ghani M, et al. Reinterpretation of sequence variants: one diagnostic laboratory's experience, and the need for standard guidelines. Genet Med 2018;20(3):365–8.
19. Rc G DL, Al M. GINA, genetic discrimination, and genomic medicine. N Engl J Med 2015;372(5):397–9.
20. Hershberger RE, Givertz MM, Ho CY, et al. Genetic Evaluation of Cardiomyopathy-A Heart Failure Society of America Practice Guideline. J Card Fail 2018;24(5):281–302.
21. Towbin JA, McKenna WJ, Abrams DJ, et al. 2019 HRS expert consensus statement on evaluation, risk stratification, and management of arrhythmogenic cardiomyopathy. Heart Rhythm 2019;16(11):e301–72.
22. Ackerman MJ, Priori SG, Willems S, et al. HRS/EHRA Expert Consensus Statement on the State of Genetic Testing for the Channelopathies and Cardiomyopathies. EP Eur 2011;13(8):1077–109.
23. Stiles MK, Wilde AAM, Abrams DJ, et al. 2020 APHRS/HRS expert consensus statement on the investigation of decedents with sudden unexplained death and patients with sudden cardiac arrest, and of their families. Heart Rhythm 2021;18(1):e1–50.
24. Verhagen JMA, Kempers M, Cozijnsen L, et al. Expert consensus recommendations on the cardiogenetic care for patients with thoracic aortic disease and their first-degree relatives. Int J Cardiol 2018;258:243–8.
25. Sturm AC, Knowles Joshua W, Gidding Samuel S, et al. Clinical Genetic Testing for Familial Hypercholesterolemia. J Am Coll Cardiol 2018;72(6):662–80.
26. Brown EE, Sturm AC, Cuchel M, et al. Genetic testing in dyslipidemia: A scientific statement from the National Lipid Association. J Clin Lipidol 2020;14(4):398–413.

Genetic Lipid Disorders Associated with Atherosclerotic Cardiovascular Disease

Molecular Basis to Clinical Diagnosis and Epidemiologic Burden

Reed Mszar, MPH[a], Gayley B. Webb, CRNP[b], Vivek T. Kulkarni, MD[b], Zahid Ahmad, MD[c], Daniel Soffer, MD[b],*

KEYWORDS

- Cardiovascular disease • Genetics • Hypercholesterolemia • Lipids
- Atherosclerosis

KEY POINTS

- The root cause of atherosclerosis is the accumulation of and response to apoB-containing lipoproteins in the subendothelium of the arterial wall balanced by the protective effects of high-density lipoprotein cholesterol (HDL-C).
- Inherited causes of lipid and lipoprotein abnormalities associated with elevated apoB and/or dysfunctional HDL are associated with premature development of atherosclerotic cardiovascular disease (ASCVD), whereas inherited causes of very low apoB-lipoproteins are associated with low lifetime risk for ASCVD.
- Identification of individuals who have specific severe inherited lipid/lipoprotein abnormalities may enable enhanced clinical attention to ASCVD risk and medical outcomes for patients and their families.
- Key features of inherited lipid/lipoprotein disorders associated with ASCVD risk are summarized for clinical reference.

[a] Yale Center for Outcomes Research and Evaluation, New Haven, CT, USA; [b] Division of Cardiovascular Medicine, Department of Medicine, Perelman School of Medicine, University of Pennsylvania, Philadelphia, PA, USA; [c] Division of Nutrition and Metabolic Disease, Department of Internal Medicine, University of Texas Southwestern Medical Center, Dallas, TX, USA
* Corresponding author. University of Pennsylvania Health System, Perelman Center for Advanced Medicine, 34th and Civic Center Boulevard, Philadelphia, PA 19104.
E-mail address: Daniel.soffer@pennmedicine.upenn.edu

Med Clin N Am 106 (2022) 325–348
https://doi.org/10.1016/j.mcna.2021.11.009
0025-7125/22/© 2021 Elsevier Inc. All rights reserved.

Abbreviations	
ABL	Abetalipoproteinemia
AP	acute pancreatitis
ApoA1	apolipoprotein A1
apoB	apolipoprotein B
ARH	Autosomal Recessive Hypercholesterolemia
ASCVD	atherosclerotic cardiovascular disease
CESD	Cholesteryl Ester Storage Disease
CM	chylomicrons
FCHL	Familial Combined Hyperlipidemia
FCS	Familial Chylomicronemia Syndrome
FDBL	Familial Dysbetalipoproteinemia
FED	Fish-Eye Disease
FHBL	Familial Hypobetalipoproteinemia
FHTG	Familial Hypertriglyceridemia
FLD	Familial LCAT Deficiency
HDL-C	high-density lipoprotein cholesterol
LCAT	Lecithin-cholesterol acyltransferase
LDL-C	low-density lipoprotein cholesterol
LDLR	low-density lipoprotein receptor
Lp(a)	Lipoprotein(a)
PAD	peripheral artery disease
PCSK9	proprotein convertase subtilisin/kexin type 9
TD	Tangier Disease
TG	triglycerides
VLDL	very low-density lipoprotein cholesterol

INTRODUCTION

Atherosclerotic cardiovascular disease (ASCVD) is a leading cause of global morbidity and mortality. Elevated levels of low-density lipoproteins (LDL) and other apolipoprotein B (apoB)-containing lipoproteins is the underlying cause of, or more precisely the substrate required for, atheroma development that precedes an ASCVD event. High-density lipoproteins (HDL) are complex units that contain lipids and a host of proteins that mostly interrupt atherogenesis and participate in other physiologic processes. The relative and absolute levels of lipoproteins and their cholesterol content are useful markers of ASCVD risk, and severe derangements in LDL cholesterol (LDL-C), apoB, non-HDL cholesterol (non-HDL-C), HDL cholesterol (HDL-C), and triglyceride (TG) levels can be defining characteristics of genetic and environmental abnormalities that predispose individuals to, or protect them from, premature ASCVD.[1] Inherited lipid and lipoprotein derangements may contribute to non-ASCVD outcomes as well, but those conditions are not the focus of this review.

Interpretation of a standard lipid profile is commonly performed as part of routine clinical practice. However, inherited lipid disorders are largely undiagnosed and undertreated in the general population. Given the importance of diagnosing disorders of lipid metabolism early in life and initiating timely and effective management with lifestyle modifications and/or pharmacotherapies to prevent and delay premature ASCVD, increased awareness of these conditions and their distinctions is critical. Furthermore, awareness of the full spectrum of inherited lipid disorders is needed because not all conditions lead to ASCVD. Rather, some may have other clinical manifestations and may be associated with reduced ASCVD risk in some cases. Accordingly, in this review, we aimed to summarize the existing literature regarding the genetics and molecular basis, clinical presentation, and epidemiologic burden of genetic lipid disorders that are associated with variations in ASCVD risk and provide clinicians with a useable resource for diagnosing and managing these conditions among their at-risk patients (**Table 1**). The following sections are grouped based on the disorder's lipid/lipoprotein concentrations and relative prevalence.

HIGH CHOLESTEROL
Common

Heterozygous familial hypercholesterolemia
Heterozygous familial hypercholesterolemia (FH) (HeFH) is a common, autosomal dominant disorder characterized by elevated LDL-C levels due to impaired LDL particle clearance. HeFH is associated with an increased risk of premature ASCVD and aortic valve stenosis.[2–4] Although effective lipid-lowering and ASCVD risk reduction can be achieved through adherence to pharmacologic therapies (eg, statins, ezetimibe, proprotein convertase subtilisin/kexin type 9 [PCSK9] inhibitors, and other agents) as well as lifestyle modifications, HeFH remains largely undetected and undertreated in the general population.[2] A formal diagnosis of HeFH may enable improved risk stratification and cascade screening of first-degree family members, thus enhancing standard of care.

Clinical presentation. The clinical diagnosis of HeFH is probabilistic and based on several weighted criteria (**Table 2**) (eg, Simon Broome, Dutch Lipid Clinic Network, and US MEDPED) that incorporate total and LDL-C concentrations, personal and family history of hypercholesterolemia and premature ASCVD, physical findings, and genetic testing results.[4] Clinicians should consider an HeFH diagnosis in adults ($\geq$20 years) with LDL-C levels greater than or equal to 190 mg/dL (4.9 mmol/L) and in children (<20 years) with LDL-C levels greater than or equal to 160 mg/dL (4.1 mmol/L), particularly given a family history of premature ASCVD and/or HeFH and in all patients with a personal history of premature ASCVD.[3] Clinical manifestations of very high LDL-C levels vary among those affected, and because extensor tendon xanthomas (Achilles, subpatellar, and hand extensor tendons) were more common in the prestatin era, genetic testing has a more important role in contemporary diagnosis (**Fig. 1**).[5] In addition to tendon xanthomas, patients with very high LDL-C levels may also present with cholesterol deposits affecting the skin of the eyelids (xanthelasmas) or the superior and inferior corneal margins (corneal arcus), although these findings may be present in other conditions as well.

Genetics and molecular basis. HeFH is caused by variations in one of 3 genes including those encoding *LDLR*, *APOB*, and *PCSK9*, resulting in inefficient LDL/LDLR (LDL receptor) interaction and impaired LDL clearance from the circulation.[6] LDL-C and ASCVD phenotypes are both determined by other factors (eg, diet, physical activity, inflammatory diseases, other environmental and genetic factors) as well, thereby leading to a wide range of LDL-C concentrations and ASCVD risk levels among those with pathogenic HeFH variants. Individuals with the HeFH lipid phenotype may have a monogenic or polygenic (see below) cause, and those with monogenic HeFH may also have polygenic risk contribution to the LDL-C level resulting in variable LDL-C levels and ASCVD risk.[7] The presence of a pathogenic variant increases ASCVD risk compared to those without an identified variant across the entire range of LDL-C from levels as low as less than 130 mg/dL to as high as greater than 220 mg/dL.[8] Individuals with monogenic HeFH have a 2- to 3.5-fold increased risk of ASCVD compared to patients with elevated LDL-C levels and no genetic variant associated with FH and more than 20-fold when comparing those with the highest LDL-C

Table 1
Overview of genetic lipid disorders' effect on lipid concentrations, molecular basis, and epidemiologic burden[69]

Genetic Lipid Disorder	Effect on Lipids	ASCVD Risk	Genes/Molecular Basis	Prevalence
High cholesterol				
Heterozygous FH	↑ LDL-C and apoB	↑	Autosomal dominant LDLR, APOB, and PCSK9	1:220–250
Polygenic hypercholesterolemia	↑ LDL-C and apoB	↑	Multiple genes with combined effect	>1:220–250
HoFH	↑ LDL-C and apoB	↑↑↑	Autosomal dominant Biallelic mutations in LDLR, APOB, and PCSK9	1:160,000–320,000
Lipoprotein(a)	↑ Lp(a) ↑ LDL-C	↑	LPA	1:7
Lysosomal acid lipase deficiency (Wolman disease or cholesteryl ester storage disease)	↑ LDL-C ↑ TG (↓ HDL-C)	↑	LIPA	1:40,000–300,000
CTX	↑ LDL-C ↑ TG	↑	Autosomal recessive CYP27A1	<1:1,000,000
Hyperalphalipoproteinemia	↑ HDL-C	↑/-/↓	CETP, SCARB1, ABCA1, and LIPC	N/A
ARH	↑ LDL-C and apoB	↑↑	Autosomal recessive LDLRAP1	1:1,000,000
Sitosterolemia	↑ LDL-C ↑ β-sitosterol	↑	Autosomal recessive ABCG5 and ABCG8	1:200,000
Low cholesterol				
Familial hypobetalipoproteinemia (or PCSK9 deficiency)	↓ ApoB ↓ LDL-C ↓ TG	→	Autosomal dominant APOB and PCSK9	1:1000–3000
Abetalipoproteinemia	↓ ApoB ↓ LDL-C ↓ TG	→	Autosomal recessive MTTP	<1:1,000,000

	Lipids	Genetics		Prevalence
Familial combined hypolipidemia	↓ ApoB ↓ LDL-C	ANGPTL3	↓	N/A
Low HDL				
TD	↓ HDL-C	Autosomal recessive ABCA1	↑/-	<1:1,000,000
FLD and FED	↓ HDL-C	Autosomal recessive LCAT	↑/-	<1:1,000,000
Apolipoprotein A1 deficiency	↓ HDL-C	Autosomal recessive APOA1	↑/↓	<1:1,000,000
High Triglycerides				
FCHL	↑ LDL-C ↑ VLDL-C ↑ apoB	Multiple genetic associations Significant environmental influence	↑↑	1:100
FDBL	↑ IDL and chylomicron remnants, normal apoB	Second hit (environmental) required APOE E2/E2 genotype	↑	1:5000
MCS	↑ chylomicrons ↑VLDL-C	Polygenic disorder	-	1:600
FHTG	↑ TG, normal apoB	Suspected autosomal dominant.	↑/-	1:100–200
FCS	↑ chylomicrons	Autosomal recessive biallelic monogenic LPL, APOC2, APOA5, GPIHBP1, LMF1, and GDP1	-	1:1,000,000
Inherited LD	↑ TG / apo	LMNA	↑/-	<1:1,000,000

Abbreviations: ABCA1, adenosine triphosphate (ATP)-binding cassette A1; ApoC2, apolipoprotein C2; ApoE, apolipoprotein E; ARH, autosomal recessive hypercholesterolemia; CETP, cholesteryl ester transfer protein; CTX, cerebrotendinous xanthomatosis; FCH, familial combined hyperlipidemia; FCS, familial chylomicronemia syndrome; FDBL, familial dysbetalipoproteinemia; FED, fish eye disease; FH, familial hypercholesterolemia; FHTG, familial hypertriglyceridemia; FLD, familial LCAT deficiency; GDP1, glyceraldehyde-3-phosphate dehydrogenase 1; GPIHBP1, glycosylphosphatidylinositol-anchored high-density lipoprotein-binding protein 1; HoFH, homozygous familial hypercholesterolemia; IDL-C, intermediate-density lipoprotein cholesterol; LCAT, lecithin-cholesterol acyltransferase; LD, lipodystrophy; LDLR, low-density lipoprotein receptor; LDLRAP1, low-density lipoprotein receptor adaptor protein 1; LIPC, hepatic lipase; LMF1, lipase maturation factor 1; Lp(a), lipoprotein(a); LPL, lipoprotein lipase; MCS, multifactorial chylomicronemia syndrome; MTTP, microsomal triglyceride transfer protein; PCSK9, proprotein convertase subtilisin/kexin type 9; SCARB1, scavenger receptor B1; TD, Tangier disease; VLDL-C, very low-density lipoprotein cholesterol; APOA1/5, apolipoprotein A1/5; ABCG5/8, ATP-binding cassette (ABC) transporters subfamily G members 5 and 8.

levels greater than 220 mg/dL with a genetic variant to individuals with normal LDL-C levels less than 130 mg/dL and no genetic variant.[8,9] The Centers for Disease Control and Prevention designates genetic testing for FH as a Tier 1 intervention, and a testing algorithm has been proposed by an international expert panel to facilitate cascade screening for individuals and families.[6]

Epidemiologic burden. HeFH affects approximately 1 in every 250 individuals worldwide, translating to as many as 34 million people globally and more than 1 million in the United States.[6] Although all races and ethnicities are impacted by HeFH, certain ancestries such as French Canadian, South African Afrikaner, Lebanese, and Ashkenazi Jewish (of Lithuanian ancestry) populations experience disproportionately higher frequencies of HeFH due to the presence of a founder effect.[10,11] Despite the readily identifiable clinical phenotype and cardiovascular risk, only 10% of those affected have been diagnosed with HeFH and even fewer receive appropriate lipid-lowering for their condition. If left untreated, affected men and women have a 30% and 50% risk of fatal or nonfatal cardiac event by 50 and 60 years of age, respectively.[6]

Polygenic hypercholesterolemia

Many individuals presenting with a phenotypic expression similar to HeFH lack an identifiable monogenic FH-associated variant, whether due to a polygenic,

Table 2
Clinical diagnostic criteria for heterozygous familial hypercholesterolemia

	US MEDPED Criteria[89]			
Age, y	First-Degree Relative With FH	Second-Degree Relative With FH	Third-Degree Relative With FH	General Population
<20	220 mg/dL (5.7 mmol/L)	230 mg/dL (5.9 mmol/L)	240 mg/dL (6.2 mmol/L)	270 mg/dL (7.0 mmol/L)
20–29	240 mg/dL (6.2 mmol/L)	250 mg/dL (6.5 mmol/L)	260 mg/dL (6.7 mmol/L)	290 mg/dL (7.5 mmol/L)
30–39	270 mg/dL (7.0 mmol/L)	280 mg/dL (7.2 mmol/L)	290 mg/dL (7.5 mmol/L)	340 mg/dL (8.8 mmol/L)
≥40	290 mg/dL (7.5 mmol/L)	300 mg/dL (7.8 mmol/L)	310 mg/dL (8.0 mmol/L)	360 mg/dL (9.3 mmol/L)

Simon Broome Criteria[90]	
Criteria	Point
Total cholesterol levels >290 mg/dL (7.5 mmol/L) or LDL-C >190 mg/dL (4.9 mmol/L) in adults. Total cholesterol levels >260 mg/dL (6.7 mmol/L) or LDL-C 155 mg/dL (4.0 mmol/L)	1
Tendon xanthomas in the patient or tendon xanthomas in a first- or second-degree relative	2
DNA-based evidence of an LDLR mutation, familial defective apo B-100, or a PCSK9 mutation	3
Family history of myocardial infarction before age 50 y in a second degree relative or before age 60 y in a first degree relative.	4
Family history of elevated total cholesterol >290 mg/dL (7.5 mmol/L) in an adult first- or second-degree relative. Family history of elevated total cholesterol >260 mg/dL (6.7 mmol/L) in a child, brother, or sister 16 y or younger	5

(continued on next page)

Table 2 (continued)	
Simon Broome Criteria[90]	
Criteria	Point
Diagnosis	*Total Score*
Definite familial hypercholesterolemia	1 + 2 or 3
Possible familial hypercholesterolemia	1 + 4 or 5
Dutch Lipid Clinic Network Criteria[91]	
Criteria	Score
Family history	
Premature CVD (men <55 y, women <60 y) in first-degree relative, OR	1
LDL >95th percentile in first-degree relative AND/OR	1
Tendon xanthoma and/or arcus cornealis in first-degree relative, OR	2
LDL >95th percentile in children <18 y	2
Personal history	
Premature CAD in patient (men <55 y, women <60 y)	2
Premature cerebral or peripheral vascular disease (men <55 y, women <60 y)	1
Clinical examination	
Tendon xanthomas, OR	6
Corneal arcus younger than 45 y	4
LDL	
>330 mg/dL (8.5 mmol/L)	8
250–329 mg/dL (6.5–8.5 mmol/L)	5
190–249 mg/dL (4.9–6.4 mmol/L)	3
155–189 mg/dL (4.0–4.9 mmol/L)	1
Presence of functional LDLR mutation (in the LDLR, ApoB, or PCSK9 gene)	8
Diagnosis based on overall score	*Total score*
Definite	>8
Probable	6–8
Possible	3–5
Unlikely	<3

Abbreviations: CAD, coronary artery disease; CVD, cardiovascular disease; LDLR, LDL receptor.

environmental, or an unknown cause.[12–14] Genetic testing to distinguish polygenic from an unknown cause is not widely available at present. It is estimated that polygenic hypercholesterolemia accounts for approximately 20% to 30% of patients with the HeFH phenotype and as high as 49% among those with severe hypercholesterolemia in the UK Biobank.[15–17] Recent evidence suggests that a higher relative LDL-C polygenic risk score was associated with an increased ASCVD risk only among individuals who also had monogenic FH.[17] Individuals should be treated based on LDL-C and ASCVD risk assessment, and treatment based on genetic screening alone is not currently recommended.[18–20]

Treatment of HeFH and polygenic hypercholesterolemia. Once HeFH and polygenic hypercholesterolemia are identified in adults, treatment should be initiated. There is more flexibility about the timing of treatment in children, but in those whose family has the highest risk for premature ASCVD, treatment may begin before 10 years of

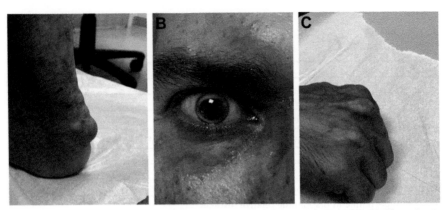

Fig. 1. Clinical findings from a patient with homozygous familial hypercholesterolemia, permission obtained. Images of (*A*) Achilles tendon xanthoma, (*B*) circumferential corneal arcus, and (*C*) metacarpal extensor tendon xanthoma.

age. In addition to a heart healthy diet low in saturated fats and dietary cholesterol, high-intensity statins are the foundation of pharmacotherapy in adults[1] and starting doses vary for each of the US Food and Drug Administration (FDA)-approved statins in children. In adults, high-potency statins (eg, rosuvastatin and atorvastatin) should be favored as the initial option. Other add-on therapies should be considered to achieve optimal LDL-C lowering, and individual thresholds can be determined by response to therapy and ASCVD risk indicators. Other add-on treatments may include ezetimibe, PCSK9 monoclonal antibodies, bile acid sequestrants, and bempedoic acid. LDL apheresis is available for individuals with HeFH who have LDL-C levels greater than or equal to 300 mg/dL or those with an LDL-C level greater than or equal to 100 mg/dL and documented coronary or peripheral artery disease (PAD).[21]

Lipoprotein(a)

Although lipoprotein(a) [Lp(a)] has long been considered a cardiovascular risk factor, its causal role in the development of premature ASCVD has received increased attention in recent years because of advancements in potential therapeutics.[22] Prospective observational studies, meta-analyses, and genome-wide association studies (GWAS) and Mendelian randomization studies have all shown that increasing plasma Lp(a) concentrations are associated with a proportional increase in the risk of coronary heart disease and aortic valve stenosis.[23–25]

Lp(a) is a plasma lipoprotein that consists of a cholesterol-rich LDL particle with an apolipoprotein B100 covalently bound to apolipoprotein(a) and high levels of oxidized phospholipids. Apolipoprotein(a) has genetic and structural homology with plasminogen, and high circulating levels may interfere with fibrinolysis and thrombolysis. Lp(a) levels are greater than 80% dictated by genetic variants that result in Kringle IV type-2 (KIV-2) copy number variation; small Lp(a) variants with few KIV-2 copies have high synthetic and reduced clearance rates resulting in high Lp(a) levels. High levels of Lp(a) are thought to contribute to ASCVD risk because of the combined effects of its LDL moiety, the antifibrinolytic effects of apo(a), and the inflammatory impact of oxidized phospholipids.

Measurement of Lp(a) is complicated by issues related to estimating risk from particle number compared to cholesterol, as well as a lack of current standardization and harmonization of international measurements. The normal distribution of Lp(a) in the general population is skewed leftward. Levels are considered either normal (less than the upper limit of normal range [30 mg/dL or 75 nmol/L]) or high. Approximately 20% of the general population has high levels, and ASCVD risk increases proportionally with Lp(a) level.

The National Lipid Association (NLA) scientific statement on the use of Lp(a) in clinical practice recommends the measurement of Lp(a) levels in adults and youth with family members who have high Lp(a) levels or premature ASCVD, and in adults with a personal history of premature clinical ASCVD, primary hypercholesterolemia, recurrent or progressive ASCVD, calcific aortic valve stenosis, or less-than-expected LDL-C reduction with statin therapy.[26] Recent randomized controlled trial evidence investigating a hepatocyte-directed antisense oligonucleotide, which inhibits the production of apolipoprotein(a), shows an achievement greater than 80% Lp(a)-lowering among patients with elevated Lp(a) levels and established ASCVD.[27] Ongoing trials are examining the impact of reducing Lp(a) on major cardiovascular events and outcomes. Otherwise, lipoprotein apheresis can be performed in adults with signs of progressive ASCVD, despite optimal medical therapy, who have LDL-C levels greater than or equal to 100 mg/dL and Lp(a) levels greater than or equal to 60 mg/dL.

Uncommon and Rare

Homozygous familial hypercholesterolemia

Homozygous FH (HoFH) is characterized by extremely high serum cholesterol levels due to LDL-C (>400 mg/dL [10.4 mmol/L]), tendon xanthomas, and a marked progression of early atherosclerosis and aortic valve stenosis (**Table 3**).[28] The diagnosis is confirmed with identification of biallelic pathogenic variants in the same genes that cause HeFH (*LDLR* or *APOB*, *PCSK9).*[28] Less severe hypercholesterolemia may be seen in individuals with compound (2 different variants of the same genetic locus [eg, inherited 2 different pathogenic variants in *LDLR*]) or double heterozygous (2 different genetic loci affected [eg, a pathogenic variants of *PCSK9* and*APOB*]) mutations. Given the severity and very early presentation of ASCVD, early detection and aggressive lipid lowering in childhood are critical for affected individuals. HoFH is rare and may impact as many as 1 in every 160,000 to 320,000 individuals, a proportion substantially higher than previously estimated (1 in 1,000,000).[2,28] It has even been shown to be as common as 1 in 30,000 in a specific Dutch Afrikaner population.[29]

Early and aggressive treatment is necessary to manage ASCVD risk. Unfortunately, LDL-C-lowering therapies are less effective for treatment of HoFH than other causes

Table 3	
Criteria for the clinical diagnosis of homozygous familial hypercholesterolemia[28]	
Clinical Criteria	**Score for Diagnosis**
1. Genetic confirmation of 2 mutant alleles at the *LDLR, APOB, PCSK9,* or *LDLRAP1* gene locus	1 or 2 + 3 or 2 + 4
2. An untreated LDL-C level >13 mmol/L (500 mg/dL) or treated LDL-C level ≥8 mmol/L (300 mg/dL)[a]	
3. Cutaneous or tendon xanthoma before age 10 y	
4. Untreated elevated LDL-C levels consistent with heterozygous FH in both patients	

Abbreviation: LDLRAP1, low-density lipoprotein receptor adaptor protein 1.

[a] LDL-C levels are indicative, and lower levels, particularly in children or in treated patients, do not exclude the presence of HoFH.

of hypercholesterolemia because those therapies rely on increasing LDLR expression. However, some individuals have enough LDLR expression to benefit from statins, ezetimibe, PCSK9 monoclonal antibodies, bile acid sequestrants, or possibly bempedoic acid, although lipoprotein apheresis is often necessary for individuals with HoFH. Lomitapide (a small molecule inhibitor of microsomal triglyceride transfer protein [MTTP]) can effectively lower LDL-C in patients with HoFH, but it is difficult to use due to fat malabsorption, steatorrhea, required low-fat diet supplemented by fat-soluble vitamins, and fatty liver as a result of its mechanism of action. In addition, evinacumab (monoclonal antibody inhibitor of angiopoietin-like protein 3 [AngPTL3]), which has a favorable safety profile, received FDA approval in February 2021 as a monthly infusion to lower LDL-C in individuals with HoFH aged 12 years or older. Both lomitapide and evinacumab can lower LDL-C in individuals who have null or near-null LDLR expression because they do not depend on LDLR activity and should be offered if standard therapies are not effective.[30] Early liver transplant is another modality that has been used for children with HoFH who do not have clinical ASCVD.[31] Investigational gene therapies and gene editing may have a role in the care of individuals with HoFH in the future.

Autosomal recessive hypercholesterolemia

Autosomal recessive hypercholesterolemia (ARH) is a rare disorder caused by biallelic pathogenic variants in the recessive low-density lipoprotein receptor adaptor protein 1 (LDLRAP1) gene, which encodes a hepatic LDLR chaperone involved in the endocytic internalization of the LDL/LDLR complex by liver cells.[32,33] Although ARH has a similar clinical presentation to HoFH, it differs as a result of its recessive mode of inheritance. The prevalence of ARH has been estimated to be approximately 1 in 1,000,000, although certain populations (Sardinia) have been shown to experience ARH at higher frequency (1:143).[34] Similar to HoFH, severe hypercholesterolemia, extensor tendon or cutaneous xanthomas, premature ASCVD, and aortic valve stenosis may be seen.[35] Among patients with ARH, LDL-C levels may be lowered up to 65% by statin monotherapy and up to 58% to 85% with combined lipid-lowering therapy using high-intensity statins and ezetimibe.[36,37] A poor cardiovascular prognosis has been observed in a recent study of 52 patients with ARH (mean follow-up: 14.1 years).[32]

Sitosterolemia

Sitosterolemia is a rare autosomal recessive disorder with features similar to HeFH characterized by the presence of tendon and tuberous xanthomas and premature ASCVD, and is associated with stomatocytosis and macrothrombocytopenia as a result of increased concentrations of phytosterols (β-sitosterol and campesterol) and LDL-C.[38,39] Biallelic pathogenic variants in the adenosine triphosphate-binding cassette (ABC) transporters, ABCG5 and ABCG8, have been shown to cause sitosterolemia.[40] Increased hepatocyte sterol levels lead to reduced LDLR expression and impaired circulatory LDL clearance.

One population-based study found that approximately 4% of individuals with LDL-C greater than or equal to 190 mg/dL have β-sitosterol concentrations greater than the 99th percentile and an estimated 0.3% had concentrations consistent with sitosterolemia.[40] Based on the study conducted by Brinton and colleagues,[40] the investigators concluded that the prevalence of sitosterolemia may be as high as 500 per million and is largely undiagnosed. The intestinal sterol absorption inhibitor, ezetimibe, is a particularly effective treatment because it reduces intestinal cholesterol and plant sterol absorption by inhibition of the Niemann-Pick C1-like 1 (NPC1L1) transporter.[41]

The diagnosis of sitosterolemia can be suggested in an individual with severe hypercholesterolemia despite absent family history and when there is blunted statin response, but an exaggerated LDL-C-lowering response to ezetimibe. The diagnosis can be confirmed by measuring plasma phytosterol composition and/or genetic confirmation.

Lysosomal acid lipase deficiency (Wolman disease or cholesteryl ester storage disorder)

Lysosomal acid lipase deficiency is a rare autosomal recessive disorder caused by biallelic pathogenic variants in the lysosomal acid lipase (*LIPA*) gene. Wolman disease is a severe disorder that presents during infancy and has an average life expectancy of less than 4 months due to liver failure, whereas cholesteryl ester storage disease (CESD) is less severe and presents later in life.[42] Both conditions are often undiagnosed or misdiagnosed as nonalcoholic fatty liver disease, nonalcoholic steatohepatitis, or cryptogenic cirrhosis because of similar features of dyslipidemia and elevated levels of transaminases. The prevalence has been estimated to be between 1:40,000 and 300,000.[42] CESD should be considered in individuals with severe hypercholesterolemia without a familial predisposition, with or without moderate hypertriglyceridemia (HTG), fatty liver disease, and liver biopsy findings of microvesicular steatosis. The diagnosis is confirmed by lysosomal acid lipase (LAL) enzyme assay and/or by genetic testing. The authors expect that expanded genetic panels used when testing for HeFH may uncover more cases of CESD. Specific treatment with enzyme replacement therapy (sebelipase alfa) is available.

Bile salt synthesis disorders

Hypercholesterolemia due to inherited disorders of the normal synthetic pathway responsible for converting hepatic cholesterol to bile salts is rare. Inherited variants leading to 7-alpha-hydroxylase deficiency have been reported, and inherited homozygous *CYP27A1* variants are associated with the rare disease, cerebrotendinous xanthomatosis. Other inherited variants in genes that regulate different steps in the bile salt synthetic pathway have been demonstrated as well and lead to high cholesterol levels, liver disease, and variable manifestations.[43,44]

High-Density Lipoprotein

Very high levels of high-density lipoprotein cholesterol (hyperalphalipoproteinemia)

Although it is widely recognized that HDL-C levels have a robust inverse relationship with ASCVD risk in observational studies, this may not be the case at extreme low and/or high HDL-C levels ($\leq$30 mg/dL or $\geq$100 mg/dL).[45,46] In fact, GWAS and Mendelian randomization studies do not demonstrate a genetic association between HDL-C and ASCVD risk.[46] In addition, specific genetic variants predisposing individuals to markedly elevated HDL-C levels, such as polymorphisms in the cholesteryl ester transfer protein (*CETP*), endothelial lipase (*LIPG*), and scavenger receptor B1 (*SCARB1*) genes, are associated with increased ASCVD risk, although findings on this association are mixed.[47–49] Furthermore, a study combining 2 prospective cohorts in the general Danish population found a significant U-shaped association between HDL-C concentrations and all-cause mortality.[50]

Given these findings, it is reasonable to conclude that the strong inverse relationship between HDL-C and ASCVD risk in the normal range is a consequence of secondary lipoprotein remodeling due to CETP and hepatic lipase activity and the direct and indirect atherosclerotic effects of TG-rich remnant lipoproteins that are in excess in those individuals, enhanced by secondary factors that typically accompany those conditions. Genetic testing for individuals with high HDL-C levels is not recommended for routine clinical care. There is no treatment directed at HDL-C levels known to reduce ASCVD risk, but if ASCVD is present, LDL-C-lowering therapy and other measures recommended for ASCVD risk reduction should be used.

LOW CHOLESTEROL
Low levels of low-density lipoprotein cholesterol/apolipoprotein B

Familial hypobetalipoproteinemia
Familial hypobetalipoproteinemia (FHBL) is an autosomal codominant lipid disorder characterized by apoB levels less than the lowest one-fifth percentile and LDL-C levels between 20 and 50 mg/dL.[51] FHBL is associated with mutations in the *APOB* (also known as [a.k.a.] FHBL-1), *PCSK9*, and *ANGPTL3* (a.k.a. FHBL-2) genes, resulting in reduced levels of serum total cholesterol, apoB, and LDL-C. More than 60 mutations resulting in truncations in *APOB* (eg, apoB2 and apoB-89) have been identified as causing FHBL along with loss-of-function mutations in *PCSK9* or *ANGPTL3*.[52] Patients with FHBL (estimated prevalence 1:1,000–3,000)[53,54] have been shown to have reduced ASCVD risk but increased risk for developing nonalcoholic fatty liver disease when associated with *APOB* variants. Heterozygous and homozygous forms of FHBL can be diagnosed from lipid profile and apoB results and confirmed with genetic testing. Making the correct diagnosis of FHBL can facilitate appropriate monitoring of liver enzymes and hepatic imaging and identification of family members with the same condition.[51,55]

Abetalipoproteinemia
Abetalipoproteinemia (ABL), or Bassen-Kornzweig syndrome, is a rare autosomal recessive disorder (estimated prevalence 1:1,000,000) identified by extremely low serum concentrations of TGs and total cholesterol (<30 mg/dL), undetectable levels of LDL-C and apoB, and the presence of fatty liver and red blood cell abnormalities, as well as potential ophthalmologic and cerebellar degeneration due to vitamin deficiencies.[51] More than 30 mutations in the *MTTP* gene have been characterized among those with ABL. Dysfunctional MTTP leads to impaired assembly of intestinally derived chylomicrons (CM) and hepatically derived very-low-density lipoproteins (VLDL), resulting in steatorrhea, fat malabsorption, and fatty liver, respectively. Early introduction of a fat-restricted diet supplemented with essential fatty acids and vitamins A and E is necessary to minimize symptoms and prevent permanent neurologic and ophthalmologic complications. Identification of the cause of this syndrome was instrumental to the conceptualization and development of lomitapide, an MTTP small molecule inhibitor, FDA-approved treatment of HoFH.

Low Levels of High-Density Lipoprotein Cholesterol (Hypoalphalipoproteinemia)

Tangier disease
Tangier disease (TD), named for the Chesapeake island where there is a clustering of affected individuals, is an extremely rare form of familial HDL deficiency characterized by serum HDL-C levels less than 5 mg/dL, extremely low levels of apolipoprotein A-I (ApoA-1; <5 mg/dL), decreased total serum cholesterol levels (<150 mg/dL), and normal or high serum TG levels. TD may manifest differently between affected patients due to the greater than 90 identified genetic mutations described previously.[56] Clinical signs vary from hyperplastic orange-yellow tonsils, anemia, peripheral neuropathy, corneal opacification, as well as hepatosplenomegaly, and are due to the accumulation of cholesteryl esters in peripheral body tissues.[57,58] TD is caused by mutations in the gene that encodes the ATP-binding cassette A1 (*ABCA1*) protein, a membrane transporter that mediates cholesterol and phospholipid efflux to lipid-poor ApoA-1 or nascent HDL.[59] Patients with TD vary in their ASCVD risk; however, carriers of *ABCA1* variants have been shown to experience a greater risk of premature

atherosclerosis.[60] To date, no specific pharmacotherapies target TD, so it is recommended that affected individuals should follow a healthy lifestyle and be monitored for the development of ASCVD and offered standard measures per national guidelines when observed.

Familial lecithin-cholesterol acyltransferase deficiency and fish eye disease

Lecithin-cholesterol acyltransferase (LCAT) deficiency is a very rare autosomal recessive disorder caused by loss-of-function mutations in the *LCAT* gene associated with both familial LCAT deficiency (FLD) and fish eye disease (FED).[61] FLD is caused by variants leading to the inactivity or absence of the LCAT enzyme, whereas FED is caused by mutations preventing LCAT from esterifying cholesterol in HDL, but not in apoB-containing lipoproteins. Consequently, relatively high levels of circulating free cholesterol in lipoprotein X (LpX; phospholipid disk complexes, loaded with free cholesterol) are observed.[62] Clinical signs of LCAT deficiency include corneal opacity (present in both FLD and FED often detected in early adulthood), hemolytic anemia, and renal disease as the primary cause of morbidity among those with FLD. Previous studies have found inconsistent associations with atherosclerotic risk.[63] Treatment options for prevention of LpX-mediated kidney damage include investigational enzyme (LCAT) replacement therapy to treat FLD.

Apolipoprotein A1 deficiency

Apolipoprotein A1 (ApoA1) deficiency is a rare, autosomal dominant disorder caused by deletions and mutations in the *APOA1* gene and characterized by the absence of the ApoA1 protein leading to extremely low HDL-C concentrations (<5 mg/dL) (with normal LDL-C and TG levels). Clinical findings vary from corneal opacities, xanthomas, and xanthelasmas to premature ASCVD and carotid atherosclerosis. A specific *APOA1* variant known as apoA1Milano, found in a small grouping of individuals from a common ancestor in Limone sul Garda, Italy, is associated with reduced ASCVD risk and prompted investigation into the now abandoned synthetic apoA1Milano as a therapeutic agent. Less often, ApoA1 deficiency can lead to neurosensory signs or manifestations of secondary amyloidosis with the potential of progressing into end-stage organ failure.[64]

HYPERTRIGLYCERIDEMIA

HTG (TG ≥ 150 mg/dL) is found in approximately 25% of the US adult population[65] and is almost always caused by a combination of environmental and inherited factors. Even in individuals with inherited HTG, environmental factors have a strong influence of TG levels and outcomes. HTG can be the result of an overproduction of TG-rich lipoproteins (TRL), excessive TG loading of TRL, ineffective peripheral hydrolysis of TG, or ineffective TRL clearance due to impaired interaction with hepatic TRL receptors. HTG confers an elevated risk of acute pancreatitis (AP) when TG levels are greater than or equal to 500 mg/dL (and especially when ≥ 2000 mg/dL), usually associated with defective TG lipolysis. ASCVD risk is more closely associated with defective TRL clearance and is manifested by elevated apoB (or non-HDL-C) levels.

Inherited HTG syndromes can be characterized according to hyperlipoproteinemia phenotype or by clinical syndrome. Historically, the classification of hyperlipidemia was based on categories described by Donald Fredrickson and colleagues in 1965 (**Table 4**).[66] However, this classification has fallen out of favor and use over time for a variety of reasons including a requirement of laboratory techniques that are no longer commercially available, variable phenotypic expression within the same individual, and the advent of alternative contemporary tools for classification of individuals based

Table 4
Frederickson classification of hyperlipoproteinemia[92]

	Frederickson Classification of Hyperlipoproteinemia		
Phenotype	Triglyceride Level	Elevated Lipoprotein	apoB
I	Severe high	CM	Low
IIa	Normal	LDL	High
IIb	Moderate high	LDL and VLDL	High
III	Moderate-severe high	TRL remnant particles	Normal
IV	Moderate-severe high	VLDL	Normal
V	Severe high	CM and VLDL	Low/normal

Abbreviation: TC, total cholesterol.

on range of lipid and lipoprotein phenotype, molecular abnormalities expected, and clinical manifestations.

In this section, we describe inherited HTG syndromes (see **Table 1**) and acknowledge that characterization of individuals based on their range of phenotypes; risks for AP and ASCVD, TG, and apoB levels; physiologic defect; and genetic cause should ultimately dictate care. Care of individuals with these syndromes should include making an accurate diagnosis and attending to environmental factors and pharmacotherapy. Genetic testing is not usually recommended for diagnosis or management because the genes that regulate TG levels tend to be recessive or expressed with variable penetrance,[20] but it may be considered in individuals with severe HTG and hyperchylomicronemia to inform prognosis, treatment plan, and expectations of pharmacologic response.

High Apolipoprotein B

Familial combined hyperlipidemia
Familial combined hyperlipidemia (FCHL) is a clinical syndrome characterized in the pregenomic era by the presence of severe hypercholesterolemia; moderate HTG; elevated apoB levels due to excess VLDL and LDL, formerly Fredrickson type IIb; along with a family history of and personal risk for premature ASCVD. There is a strong association with other cardiometabolic risk factors including abdominal obesity, insulin resistance/diabetes mellitus, fatty liver, and elevated TG and reduced HDL-C levels. This common condition has an estimated prevalence in the general population of 1:100.[67–69] Multiple genetic markers have been associated with FCHL, and some individuals may have HeFH plus additional inherited or acquired predisposition to HTG. There is no genetic profile specific to FCHL. Although this is not a distinct genetic syndrome per se, the clinical finding of an individual with features of FCHL warrants attentive care to mitigate ASCVD risk. There are no specific guidelines for the management of FCHL, but high-intensity statin therapy should be the foundation of care in accordance with recommendations for treatment of primary hyperlipidemia, and additional non-HDL-C and apoB treatment targets should be tailored to individual needs and according to contemporary guidelines.[1,70–72]

Normal or Low Apolipoprotein B

Familial dysbetalipoproteinemia
Familial dysbetalipoproteinemia (FDBL), previously referred to as Fredrickson type III hyperlipoproteinemia, is characterized by elevated serum levels of remnant particles

due to dysfunctional apolipoprotein E (apoE), low or normal apoB levels, and greater ASCVD risk.[73,74] ApoE is the principal ligand for the hepatic lipoprotein remnant receptor and is a secondary ligand for the LDLR. Common and rare variants in *APOE* are associated with dysbetalipoproteinemia. There are 3 common (wild-type) *APOE* alleles, referred to as ε3, ε4, and ε2 (in order of most to least common) that dictate apoE expression. ApoE3 is considered the "parent form," apoE2 is expressed as a result of a single amino acid substitution Arg158Cys near the LDL recognition site on the gene locus, and apoE4 is expressed because of a different amino acid substitution Cys112Arg, which impairs VLDL lipolysis.[75] As a result, individuals may inherit homozygous or heterozygous combinations of the 3 common alleles in any of 6 combinations, and a meta-analysis that examined the influence of genotype on lipid levels found a linear relationship between LDL-C and ASCVD risk in the following ascending order (ε2/ε2, ε2/ε3, ε2/ε4; ε3/ε3, ε3/ε4, ε4/ε4) and that only the ε2/ε2 genotype was associated with elevated TG levels.[76] Although apoE2/E2 is the most common cause, rare genetic variants in *APOE* have also been associated with dysbetalipoproteinemia.[73] The genetic predisposition is not sufficient to manifest hyperlipidemia, however, and susceptible individuals may have normal or even low lipid levels most or all of their life until there is metabolic stress causing increased hepatic VLDL overproduction.

Common secondary factors that enhance hepatic VLDL production such as medications, alcohol intake, diet, abdominal obesity and weight gain, insulin resistance/diabetes mellitus, hypothyroidism, pregnancy, or other hormonal triggers act as a "second hit" triggering severe hyperlipidemia, which may be accompanied by xanthomas (eruptive, tuberous, or palmar) and ASCVD (especially peripheral arterial disease). Severe HTG and AP may also occur. Consequently, individuals with FDBL may have a normal measured lipid profile and then develop sudden moderate-severe combined hyperlipidemia, characterized by TG to total cholesterol ratio (TG:TC) less than 3:1 as a result of excess intermediate-density lipoprotein (IDL) levels.

LDL-C estimates by the Friedewald equation or Martin-Hopkins methods are not accurate, and detergent methods of measuring LDL-C levels directly have not been evaluated in FDBL. The defining lipid-lipoprotein tool for confirmation of remnant excess is beta-quantification or gel electrophoresis from ultracentrifugation demonstrating high VLDL-C:TG greater than 0.69 has been replaced by patterns of total cholesterol, TG, and apoB levels characterized by Allan Sniderman and colleagues[77] and confirmed by apoE genotyping. In addition to lifestyle modifications to address the environmental triggers, pharmacologic management should begin with fibrates, and then may include a combination of high-dose omega-3 fatty acid supplementation and statins.[69]

Familial hypertriglyceridemia

Familial hypertriglyceridemia (FHTG), previously referred to as Fredrickson type IV hyperlipoproteinemia, is a syndrome historically characterized by persistent moderate-severe HTG due to excess VLDL, low HDL-C, and LDL-C levels; normal apoB levels; a family history of HTG; and variable risk for ASCVD or AP. Although this seems to have a dominant inheritance pattern, it is now recognized that individuals with FHTG have a polygenic cause with a high degree of environmental sensitivity and thus a wide range of TG levels throughout their lifetime. Similar to the aforementioned conclusions about FCHL that there is clinical utility in the identification of an individual based on clinical syndrome, even though there is not a singular underlying cause, identification of individuals with features of FHTG is noteworthy. Lifetime AP and ASCVD risk are proportional to TG and apoB levels, respectively, and treatment should be customized to individual needs and applied based on national guideline recommendations of care to reduce ASCVD and AP risk.[78]

Multifactorial chylomicronemia syndrome

Multifactorial chylomicronemia syndrome (MCS), previously referred to as Fredrickson type V hyperlipoproteinemia, is a polygenic disorder often due to heterozygous variants of the lipoprotein lipase gene[79] and its important cofactors, is highly sensitive to environmental conditions (especially obesity, weight gain, dietary stressors, alcohol, medications, endocrinopathies), and characterized by severe HTG due to VLDL and CM excess. Similar to questions raised earlier about whether FCHL and FHTG should be considered distinct syndromes, individuals with features of MCS represent the far end of the HTG spectrum due to polygenic and environmental causes. In that respect, an individual with FHTG may manifest persistent VLDL excess (moderate-severe) and then transform to VLDL/CM excess (very severe HTG) due to environmental stress (eg, diet change, weight gain, development of insulin resistance and diabetes, other endocrinologic conditions, medications, alcohol excess).

Reversal of environmental stressors may enable return to the previous moderate HTG in these individuals. Thus, it is important to distinguish whether individuals presenting with severe HTG have MCS or familial chylomicronemia syndrome (FCS, see later). A European working group has created a clinical score to help distinguish MCS from FCS without the need for genetic testing, although this score still requires validation in diverse populations.[79–81]

Low Apolipoprotein B

Familial chylomicronemia syndrome

FCS, previously referred to as Fredrickson type 1 hyperlipoproteinemia, is a rare (1:1,000,000) autosomal recessive disorder caused by biallelic pathogenic variants in genes that code for lipoprotein lipase (LPL) or its cofactors (APOC2, APOA5, LMF1, GPIHBP1) leading to persistently low LPL activity.[82] Approximately 80% of FCS cases are related to mutations in LPL, previously referred to as lipoprotein lipase deficiency (LPLD), for which 180 distinct mutations have been identified.[83] Fasting serum TG levels tend to persist greater than 880 mg/dL (10 mmol/L) (**Table 5**).[71,82,84]

Elevated levels of circulating CM in MCS and FCS can lead to eruptive xanthomas or lipemia retinalis (in the retinal blood vessels). Hyperchylomicronemia is associated with increased risk of recurrent episodes of abdominal pain or even severe/recurrent AP, a life-threatening complication with overall mortality rates between 5% and 6%.[85,86] Compared with patients with HTG attributed to other conditions, those affected by chylomicronemia due to biallelic pathogenic LPL genetic variants are at a significantly greater risk for pancreatitis.[85] Premature ASCVD risk in individuals with FCS is not expected, although late-onset ASCVD may occur due to other provoking factors (eg, smoking, diabetes mellitus). Contemporary HTG pharmacotherapy tends to be ineffective for patients with FCS who have very low or no LPL activity. Novel investigational products that lower TG levels by targeting apolipoprotein C-III (ApoC-III) show promise for the care of patients with FCS. Use of the MTTP inhibitor, lomitapide, has been proposed as pharmacologic treatment of FCS, but is not recommended or available for use because of unacceptable side effects (eg, steatorrhea and hepatic steatosis) and restrictive FDA approval as therapy for HoFH. Orlistat, an intestinal lipase inhibitor has also been proposed as pharmacologic therapy for FCS as an adjunct to dietary modification directed at inhibiting CM production by severely limiting fat consumption to 15 to 20 g/d[82,87]

Inherited Lipodystrophy

Inherited lipodystrophy (LD) syndromes are characterized as conditions in which there is abnormal body fat distribution resulting in clinically significant metabolic

Table 5
Classification of hypertriglyceridemia based on the 3 internationally recognized clinical guidelines[92]

ESC/EAS Guidelines for the Management of Dyslipidemias, 2019[72]		
	Serum Triglyceride Concentration	
Normal	<1.7 mmol/L	<150 mg/dL
Moderate	1.7–9.9 mmol/L	150–880 mg/dL
Severe	>10 mmol/L	>880 mg/dL
AHA/ACC/Multisociety Guideline on the Management of Blood Cholesterol, 2018[1]		
Normal	≤2.0 mmol/L	≤175 mg/dL
Mild-moderate	2.0–5.6 mmol/L	175–499 mg/dL
Severe	≥5.7 mmol/L	≥500 mg/dL
The Endocrine Society Clinical Practice Guideline on the Evaluation and Treatment of Hypertriglyceridemia, 2012[92,a]		
Normal	<1.7 mmol/L	<150 mg/dL
Mild hypertriglyceridemia	1.7–2.3 mmol/L	150–199 mg/dL
Moderate hypertriglyceridemia	2.3–11.2 mmol/L	200–999 mg/dL
Severe hypertriglyceridemia	11.2–22.4 mmol/L	1000–1999 mg/dL
Very severe hypertriglyceridemia	≥22.4 mmol/L	≥2000 mg/dL

[a] The criteria developed for The Endocrine Society (2010) guidelines focus on the ability to assess risk for premature cardiovascular disease versus risk for pancreatitis. Presence of mild or moderate hypertriglyceridemia is commonly due to a dominant underlying cause in each patient, whereas severe or very severe hypertriglyceridemia is likely due to multiple contributing factors.[92]

derangements especially insulin resistance, fatty liver, HTG, and muscular hypertrophy in subtypes as well. There are both acquired and inherited LD syndromes, and these may result in generalized or partial loss of peripheral adipose. Inherited syndromes are classified by body morphology and the most common cause of partial LD, Donnegan type, has discrete monogenic causes (most commonly associated with *LMNA* variants), whereas other types are associated with polygenic or unknown causes. In addition to a wide range of reduced leptin levels, leptin resistance may be seen. Detailed descriptions of LD syndromes are found elsewhere, and readers are encouraged to familiarize themselves to enable earlier recognition.[88]

Genetic testing to confirm specific LD syndromes is useful but not necessary in the management of care for affected individuals and their families. However, confirmation of a diagnosis can have profound psychological benefit to affected individuals. In addition to care provided for the metabolic derangements, attention to the psychological needs of patients who experience significant body image distortion, is strongly recommended.

Underlying defects in peripheral adipose expression seen in LD syndromes result in impaired peripheral lipolysis and fatty acid mobilization, causing elevated serum TG levels due to delayed catabolism and increased hepatic TG neogenesis. TG and apoB levels may range from moderate to severely elevated. Normal therapeutic strategies for management of insulin resistance, hyperglycemia, fatty liver, ASCVD, and HTG should be used. In the case of generalized LD and leptin deficiency, synthetic leptin replacement therapy may enable optimization of these parameters as well as insatiable hunger when present and is being investigated as a treatment for partial LD at present.

SUMMARY

Together, genetic lipid disorders, ranging from common dyslipidemias such as HeFH, Lp(a), and familial combined hyperlipidemia to rare disorders including familial chylomicronemia syndrome and inherited hypoalphalipoproteinemias (ie, TD and FED), affect millions of individuals in the United States and tens of millions around the world and are often left undetected and undertreated in the general population.

Although hyperlipidemia is generally considered an important cause of ASCVD and hypolipidemia is considered protective, inherited syndromes have specific risks for this condition. HoFH has the highest ASCVD risk of all the inherited conditions, followed by FCHL, HeFH, Lp(a), and other rare disorders associated with high LDL-C and apoB. HTG syndromes are more closely associated with AP risk than ASCVD, although FDBL is associated with higher PAD risk and individuals with MCS tend to have high ASCVD risk associated primarily with comorbidities that increase TG levels and ASCVD risk factors like obesity and diabetes mellitus.

Although HDL-C is widely recognized as having an inverse relationship with ASCVD risk, at the severe ends of the HDL-C spectrum, both severe elevations and reductions may be associated with ASCVD risk in a U-shaped pattern. Low cholesterol syndromes are otherwise associated with lower ASCVD risk and are primarily worth recognizing due to other medical concerns associated with these conditions and as inherited models that may inform investigation into apoB-reducing pharmacotherapies.

Genetic testing for individuals with the HeFH phenotype, a common dominant trait, enables identification of at-risk family members and may lead to enhanced care for individuals affected by this condition. Genetic testing may have a role in the clinical care of patients with severe HTG/hyperchylomicronemia as well including when FDBL is suspected. Investigational therapies that target regulators of lipid metabolism, enzyme replacement therapy, gene therapy, and gene editing show promise for the management of inherited lipid disorders when conventional therapies may be inadequate.

CLINICS CARE POINTS

- Clinicians should be alert for the potential of an inherited lipid disorder or syndrome when severe derangements in lipid parameters are found.

- Identification of secondary environmental factors should be considered and managed accordingly before reaching conclusions about the relative impact of inherited characteristics.

- In addition to a standard lipid profile, apoB (and apoA1 in the hypoalphalipoproteinemia syndromes) should be tested to help make the diagnosis.

- ASCVD risk evaluation should be performed and syndromic risk considered when managing care.

- Genetic testing has an important role in informing ASCVD risk prognosis in the HeFH phenotype, distinguishing it from rare disorders which require specific therapy, and enabling cascade screening of family members when a dominant trait is found.

- Genetic testing has a limited role in HTG but may be used to differentiate FCS from MCS to inform therapy and confirm the diagnosis of FDBL.

DISCLOSURES

R. Mszar, G.B. Webb, V.T. Kulkarni: none. Z. Ahmad: consultant fees from Akcea Therapeutics and Esperion. D. Soffer: has received consultant fees from Akcea

Therapeutics and Novartis and institutional support for participation in clinical trials with Amgen, AstraZeneca, Ionis, Novartis, Regeneron, REGENXBIO.

REFERENCES

1. Grundy SM, Stone NJ, Bailey AL, et al. 2018 AHA/ACC/AACVPR/AAPA/ABC/ACPM/ADA/AGS/APhA/ASPC/NLA/PCNA guideline on the Management of Blood Cholesterol: A Report of the American College of Cardiology/American Heart Association Task Force on clinical practice guidelines. Circulation 2019;139:e1082–143.

2. Nordestgaard BG, Chapman MJ, Humphries SE, et al. Familial hypercholesterolaemia is underdiagnosed and undertreated in the general population: guidance for clinicians to prevent coronary heart disease: consensus statement of the European Atherosclerosis Society. Eur Heart J 2013;34:3478–3490a.

3. Gidding SS, Champagne MA, de Ferranti SD, et al. The Agenda for Familial Hypercholesterolemia: A Scientific Statement From the American Heart Association. Circulation 2015;132:2167–92.

4. McGowan MP, Hosseini Dehkordi SH, Moriarty PM, et al. Diagnosis and Treatment of Heterozygous Familial Hypercholesterolemia. J Am Heart Assoc 2019; 8:e013225.

5. Bermudez EB, Storey L, Mayo S, et al. An Unusual Case of Multiple Tendinous Xanthomas Involving the Extremities and the Ears. Case Rep Dermatol 2015; 7(3):340–4.

6. Sturm AC, Knowles JW, Gidding SS, et al. Clinical genetic testing for familial hypercholesterolemia: JACC Scientific Expert Panel. J Am Coll Cardiol 2018;72(6): 662–80.

7. Trinder M, Paquette M, Cermakova L, et al. Polygenic contribution to low-density lipoprotein cholesterol levels and cardiovascular risk in monogenic familial hypercholesterolemia. Circ Genom Precis Med 2020;13(5):515–23.

8. Khera AV, Won HH, Peloso GM, et al. Diagnostic Yield and Clinical Utility of Sequencing Familial Hypercholesterolemia Genes in Patients With Severe Hypercholesterolemia. J Am Coll Cardiol 2016;67(22):2578–89.

9. Tada H, Kawashiri MA, Nohara A, et al. Impact of clinical signs and genetic diagnosis of familial hypercholesterolaemia on the prevalence of coronary artery disease in patients with severe hypercholesterolaemia. Eur Heart J 2017;38(20):1573–9.

10. Austin MA, Hutter CM, Zimmern RL, et al. Genetic Causes of Monogenic Heterozygous Familial Hypercholesterolemia: A HuGE Prevalence Review. Am J Epidemiol 2004;160:407–20.

11. Mszar R, Buscher S, Taylor HL, et al. Familial Hypercholesterolemia and the Founder Effect Among Franco-Americans: A Brief History and Call to Action. CJC Open 2020;2:161–7.

12. Clarke RE, Padayachee ST, Preston R, et al. Effectiveness of alternative strategies to define index case phenotypes to aid genetic diagnosis of familial hypercholesterolaemia. Heart 2013;99(3):175–80.

13. Damgaard D, Larsen ML, Nissen PH, et al. The relationship of molecular genetic to clinical diagnosis of familial hypercholesterolemia in a Danish population. Atherosclerosis 2005;180(1):155–60.

14. Trinder M, Francis GA, Brunham LR. Association of monogenic vs polygenic hypercholesterolemia with risk of atherosclerotic cardiovascular disease. JAMA Cardiol 2020;5(4):390–9.

15. Wang J, Dron JS, Ban MR, et al. Polygenic versus monogenic causes of hyper-cholesterolemia ascertained clinically. Arterioscler Thromb Vasc Biol 2016; 36(12):2439–45.

16. Talmud PJ, Shah S, Whittall R, et al. Use of low-density lipoprotein cholesterol gene score to distinguish patients with polygenic and monogenic familial hyper-cholesterolaemia: a case-control study. Lancet 2013;381(9874):1293–301.

17. Trinder M, Li X, DeCastro ML, et al. Risk of premature atherosclerotic disease in patients with monogenic versus polygenic familial hypercholesterolemia. J Am Coll Cardiol 2019;74(4):512–22.

18. Mszar R, Nasir K, Santos RD. Coronary Artery Calcification in Familial Hypercho-lesterolemia: An Opportunity for Risk Assessment and Shared Decision Making With the Power of Zero? Circulation 2020;142(15):1405–7.

19. Mszar R, Grandhi GR, Valero-Elizondo J, et al. Absence of Coronary Artery Calci-fication in Middle Aged Familial Hypercholesterolemia Patients Without Athero-sclerotic Cardiovascular Disease. J Am Coll Cardiol Img 2020;13:1090–2.

20. Brown EE, Sturm AC, Cuchel M, et al. Genetic testing in dyslipidemia: A scientific statement from the National Lipid Association. J Clin Lipidol 2020;14(4):398–413.

21. Letter dated April 21, 2020; Re: P910018/S027 Trade/Device Name: LIPO-SORBER LA-15 System Product Code: MMY Filed: August 15, 2019 Amended: January 22, 2020, April 8, 2020.

22. Nordestgaard BG, Chapman MJ, Ray K, et al. Lipoprotein(a) as a cardiovascular risk factor: current status. Eur Heart J 2010;31(23):2844–53.

23. Erqou S, Kaptoge S, Perry PL, et al. Emerging Risk Factors Collaboration. Lipo-protein(a) concentration and the risk of coronary heart disease, stroke, and nonvascular mortality. JAMA 2009;302(4):412–23.

24. Nordestgaard BG, Langsted A. Lipoprotein (a) as a cause of cardiovascular dis-ease: insights from epidemiology, genetics, and biology. J Lipid Res 2016;57(11): 1953–75.

25. Clarke R, Peden JF, Hopewell JC, et al. Genetic variants associated with Lp(a) lipoprotein level and coronary disease. N Engl J Med 2009;361(26):2518–28.

26. Wilson DP, Jacobson TA, Jones PH, et al. Use of Lipoprotein(a) in clinical prac-tice: A biomarker whose time has come. A scientific statement from the National Lipid Association. J Clin Lipidol 2019;13(3):374–92.

27. Tsimikas S, Karwatowska-Prokopczuk E, Gouni-Berthold I, et al. Lipoprotein(a) Reduction in Persons with Cardiovascular Disease. N Engl J Med 2020;382(3): 244–55.

28. Cuchel M, Bruckert E, Ginsberg HN, et al. Homozygous familial hypercholester-olaemia: new insights and guidance for clinicians to improve detection and clin-ical management. A position paper from the Consensus Panel on Familial Hypercholesterolaemia of the European Atherosclerosis Society. Eur Heart J 2014;35:2146–57.

29. Seftel HC, Baker SG, Sandler MP, et al. A host of hypercholesterolaemic homozy-gotes in South Africa. Br Med J 1980;281:633–6.

30. Raal FJ, Rosenson RS, Reeskamp LF, et al. Evinacumab for Homozygous Familial Hypercholesterolemia. N Engl J Med 2020;383(8):711–20.

31. Ishigaki Y, Kawagishi N, Hasegawa Y, et al. Liver Transplantation for Homozygous Familial Hypercholesterolemia. J Atheroscler Thromb 2019;26(2):121–7.

32. D'Erasmo L, Minicocci I, Nicolucci A, et al. Autosomal Recessive Hypercholester-olemia: Long-Term Cardiovascular Outcomes. J Am Coll Cardiol 2018;71(3): 279–88.

33. Garuti R, Jones C, Li WP, et al. The modular adaptor protein autosomal recessive hypercholesterolemia (ARH) promotes low density lipoprotein receptor clustering into clathrin-coated pits. J Biol Chem 2005;280(49):40996–1004.

34. Sniderman AD, Tsimikas S, Fazio S. The severe hypercholesterolemia phenotype: clinical diagnosis, management, and emerging therapies. J Am Coll Cardiol 2014;63(19):1935–47.

35. Sanchez-Hernandez RM, Prieto-Matos P, Civeira F, et al. Autosomal recessive hypercholesterolemia in Spain. Atherosclerosis 2018;269:1–5.

36. Fellin R, Arca M, Zuliani G, et al. The history of Autosomal Recessive Hypercholesterolemia (ARH). From clinical observations to gene identification. Gene 2015; 555(1):23–32.

37. Lind S, Olsson AG, Eriksson M, et al. Autosomal recessive hypercholesterolaemia: normalizationof plasma LDL cholesterol by ezetimibe in combinationwith statin treatment. J Intern Med 2004;256:406–12.

38. Lee M-H, Lu K, Patel SB. Genetic basis of sitosterolemia. Curr Opin Lipidol 2001; 12:141–9.

39. Xu L, Wen W, Yang Y, et al. Features of Sitosterolemia in Children. Am J Cardiol 2020;125(9):1312–6.

40. Brinton EA, Hopkins PN, Hegele RA, et al. The association between hypercholesterolemia and sitosterolemia, and report of a sitosterolemia kindred. J Clin Lipidol 2018;12(1):152–61.

41. Davis HR Jr, Zhu LJ, Hoos LM, et al. Niemann-Pick C1 Like 1 (NPC1L1) is the intestinal phytosterol and cholesterol transporter and a key modulator of whole-body cholesterol homeostasis. J Biol Chem 2004;279(32):33586–92.

42. Pericleous M, Kelly C, Wang T, et al. Wolman's disease and cholesteryl ester storage disorder: the phenotypic spectrum of lysosomal acid lipase deficiency. Lancet Gastroenterol Hepatol 2017;2(9):670–9.

43. Pullinger CR, Eng C, Salen G, et al. Human cholesterol 7alpha-hydroxylase (CYP7A1) deficiency has a hypercholesterolemic phenotype. J Clin Invest 2002;110(1):109–17.

44. Chiang JYL, Ferrell JM. Up to date on cholesterol 7 alpha-hydroxylase (CYP7A1) in bile acid synthesis. Liver Res 2020;4(2):47–63.

45. Landmesser U, Hazen S. HDL-cholesterol, genetics, and coronary artery disease: the myth of the 'good cholesterol. Eur Heart J 2018;39(23):2179–82.

46. Rosenson RS, Brewer HB Jr, Barter PJ, et al. HDL and atherosclerotic cardiovascular disease: genetic insights into complex biology. Nat Rev Cardiol 2018; 15(1):9–19.

47. Agerholm-Larsen B, Nordestgaard BG, Steffensen R, et al. Elevated HDL cholesterol is a risk factor for ischemic heart disease in white women when caused by a common mutation in the cholesteryl ester transfer protein gene. Circulation 2000; 101:1907–12.

48. Johannsen TH, Frikke-Schmidt R, Schou J, et al. Genetic inhibition of CETP, ischemic vascular disease and mortality, and possible adverse effects. J Am Coll Cardiol 2012;60(20):2041–8.

49. Andersen RV, Wittrup HH, Tybjærg-Hansen A, et al. Hepatic lipase mutations,elevated high-density lipoprotein cholesterol, and increased risk of ischemic heart disease. J Am Coll Cardiol 2003;41(11):1972–82.

50. Madsen CM, Varbo A, Nordestgaard BG. Extreme high high-density lipoprotein cholesterol is paradoxically associated with high mortality in men and women: two prospective cohort studies. Eur Heart J 2017;38(32):2478–86.

51. Welty FK. Hypobetalipoproteinemia and abetalipoproteinemia: liver disease and cardiovascular disease. Curr Opin Lipidol 2020;31(2):49–55.

52. Burnett JR, Bell DA, Hooper AJ, et al. Clinical utility gene card for: Familial hypo-betalipoproteinaemia (APOB)–Update 2014. Eur J Hum Genet 2015;23(6). https://doi.org/10.1038/ejhg.2014.225.

53. Tarugi P, Averna M, Di Leo E, et al. Molecular diagnosis of hypobetalipoproteine-mia: an ENID review. Atherosclerosis 2007;195(2):e19–27.

54. Cariou B, Challet-Bouju G, Bernard C, et al. Prevalence of hypobetalipoproteine-mia and related psychiatric characteristics in a psychiatric population: results from the retrospective HYPOPSY Study. Lipids Health Dis 2018;17(1):249.

55. Pelusi S, Baselli G, Pietrelli A, et al. Rare Pathogenic Variants Predispose to He-patocellular Carcinoma in Nonalcoholic Fatty Liver Disease. Sci Rep 2019;9(1): 3682.

56. Rhyne J, Mantaring MM, Gardner DF, et al. Multiple splice defects in ABCA1 cause low HDL-C in a family with hypoalphalipoproteinemia and premature cor-onary disease. BMC Med Genet 2009;10:1.

57. Puntoni M, Sbrana F, Bigazzi F, et al. Tangier Disease. Am J Cardiovasc Drugs 2012;12:303–11.

58. Negi SI, Brautbar A, Virani SS, et al. A novel mutation in the ABCA1 gene causing an atypical phenotype of Tangier disease. J Clin Lipidol 2013;7(1):82–7.

59. Tang C, Oram JF. The cell cholesterol exporter ABCA1 as a protector from cardio-vascular disease and diabetes. Biochim Biophys Acta 2009;1791(7):563–72.

60. Asztalosa BF, Brousseaua ME, McNamaraa JR, et al. Subpopulations of high density lipoproteins in homozygous and heterozygous Tangier disease. Athero-sclerosis 2001;156:217–25.

61. Pavanello C, Calabresi L. Genetic, biochemical, and clinical features of LCAT deficiency: update for 2020. Curr Opin Lipidol 2020;31(4):232–7.

62. Jonas A. Lecithin cholesterol acyltransferase. Biochim Biophys Acta 2000;1529: 245–56.

63. Oldoni F, Baldassarre D, Castelnuovo S, et al. Complete and Partial Lecithin:Cho-lesterol Acyltransferase Deficiency Is Differentially Associated With Atheroscle-rosis. Circulation 2018;138(10):1000–7.

64. Santos RD, Schaefer EJ, Asztalos BF, et al. Characterization of high density lipo-protein particles in familial apolipoprotein A-I deficiency. J Lipid Res 2008;49(2): 349–57.

65. Carroll MD, Kit BK, Lacher DA. Trends in elevated triglyceride in adults: United States, 2001–2012. NCHS data brief, no 198. Hyattsville (MD): National Center for Health Statistics; 2015.

66. Fredrickson DS, Lees RS. A system for phenotyping hyperlipoproteinemia. Circu-lation 1965;31:321–7.

67. Hopkins PN, Heiss G, Ellison RC, et al. Coronary artery disease risk in familial combined hyperlipidemia and familial hypertriglyceridemia: a case-control com-parison from the National Heart, Lung, and Blood Institute Family Heart Study. Cir-culation 2003;108(5):519–23.

68. Veerkamp MJ, Graaf Jd, Bredie SJ, et al. Diagnosis of familial combined hyper-lipidemia based on lipid phenotype expression in 32 families: results of a 5-year follow-up study. Arterioscler Thromb Vasc Biol 2002;22:274–82.

69. Catapano AL, Graham I, De Backer G, et al. 2016 ESC/EAS guidelines for the management of dyslipidaemias. Atherosclerosis 2016;253:281–344.

70. van Greevenbroek MM, Stalenhoef AF, de Graaf J, et al. Familial combined hyper-lipidemia: from molecular insights to tailored therapy. Curr Opin Lipidol 2014; 25(3):176–82.

71. Hegele RA, Ginsberg HN, Chapman MJ, et al. The polygenic nature of hypertri-glyceridaemia: implications for definition, diagnosis, and management. Lancet Diabetes Endocrinol 2014;2(8):655–66.

72. Mach F, Baigent C, Catapano AL, et al. 2019 ESC/EAS Guidelines for the man-agement of dyslipidaemias: lipid modification to reduce cardiovascular risk. Eur Heart J 2020;41(1):111–88.

73. Koopal C, Marais AD, Visseren FL. Familial dysbetalipoproteinemia: an under-diagnosed lipid disorder. Curr Opin Endocrinol Diabetes Obes 2017;24(2):133–9.

74. Nordestgaard BG. Triglyceride-Rich Lipoproteins and Atherosclerotic Cardiovas-cular Disease: New Insights From Epidemiology, Genetics, and Biology. Circ Res 2016;118(4):547–63.

75. Phillips MC. Apolipoprotein E isoforms and lipoprotein metabolism. IUBMB Life 2014;66(9):616–23.

76. Bennet AM, Angelantonio ED, Ye Z, et al. Association of apolipoprotein E geno-types with lipid levels and coronary risk. JAMA 2007;298(11):1300–11.

77. Sniderman AD, de Graaf J, Thanassoulis G, et al. The spectrum of type III hyper-lipoproteinemia. J Clin Lipidol 2018;12(6):1383–9.

78. Laufs U, Parhofer KG, Ginsberg HN, et al. Clinical review on triglycerides. Eur Heart J 2020;41(1):99–109c.

79. Moulin P, Dufour R, Averna M, et al. Identification and diagnosis of patients with familial chylomicronaemia syndrome (FCS): Expert panel recommendations and proposal of an "FCS score. Atherosclerosis 2018;275:265–72.

80. Paquette M, Bernard S, Hegele RA, et al. Chylomicronemia: Differences between familial chylomicronemia syndrome and multifactorial chylomicronemia. Athero-sclerosis 2019;283:137–42.

81. O'Dea LSL, MacDougall J, Alexander VJ, et al. Differentiating Familial Chylomi-cronemia Syndrome From Multifactorial Severe Hypertriglyceridemia by Clinical Profiles. J Endocr Soc 2019;3(12):2397–410.

82. Stroes E, Moulin P, Parhofer KG, et al. Diagnostic algorithm for familial chylomi-cronemia syndrome. Atheroscler Suppl 2017;23:1–7.

83. Rabacchi C, Pisciotta L, Cefalu AB, et al. Spectrum of mutations of the LPL gene identified in Italy in patients with severe hypertriglyceridemia. Atherosclerosis 2015;241(1):79–86.

84. Chait A, Brunzell JD. Chylomicronemia syndrome. Adv Intern Med 1991;37: 249–73.

85. Valdivielso P, Ramírez-Bueno A, Ewald N. Current knowledge of hypertriglyceri-demic pancreatitis. Eur J Intern Med 2014;25(8):689–94.

86. Whitcomb DC. Acute Pancreatitis. N Engl J Med 2006;354:2142–50.

87. Williams L, Rhodes KS, Karmally W, et al. patients, families living with FCS. Famil-ial chylomicronemia syndrome: Bringing to life dietary recommendations throughout the life span. J Clin Lipidol 2018;12(4):908–19.

88. Akinci B, Sahinoz M, Oral E. Lipodystrophy Syndromes: Presentation and Treat-ment. In: Feingold KR, Anawalt B, Boyce A, et al, editors. Endotext. South Dart-mouth (MA): MDText.com, Inc.; 2018. p. 2000. Available at: https://www.ncbi.nlm.nih.gov/books/NBK513130/.

89. Williams RR, Hunt SC, Schumacher MC, et al. Diagnosing Heterozygous Familial Hypercholesterolemia Using New Practical Criteria Validated by Molecular Ge-netics. Am J Cardiol 1993;72:171–6.

90. Scientific Steering Committee on behalf of the Simon Broome Register Group. Risk of fatal coronary heart disease in familial hypercholesterolaemia. BMJ 1991;303:893–6.

91. World Health Organization. Familial hypercholesterolemia—report of a second WHO Consultation. Geneva (Switzerland): World Health Organization; 1999. WHO publication no. WHO/HGN/FH/CONS/99.2).

92. Berglund L, Brunzell JD, Goldberg AC, et al. Endocrine s. Evaluation and treatment of hypertriglyceridemia: an Endocrine Society clinical practice guideline. J Clin Endocrinol Metab 2012;97(9):2969–89.

Cardio-Rheumatology
Prevention of Cardiovascular Disease in Inflammatory Disorders

Paul Nona, MD, Cori Russell, MD*

KEYWORDS

- Inflammation • Prevention • Rheumatoid arthritis • Systemic lupus erythematosus
- Cardiovascular disease

KEY POINTS

- Patients with chronic inflammatory conditions are at increased risk of cardiovascular disease.
- Traditional risk assessment tools underestimate risk of cardiovascular disease in this patient population.
- Clinicians should consider the use of additional cardiovascular disease screening tools, such as disease-specific risk calculators and subclinical atherosclerosis imaging.
- Multidisciplinary teams can improve preventive cardiac care in patients with underlying chronic inflammatory conditions.

INTRODUCTION

Inflammation plays a well-established role in the development and progression of atherosclerosis.[1,2] Individuals with underlying chronic inflammatory conditions are at increased risk of developing cardiovascular disease, including coronary artery disease and heart failure (**Fig. 1**). Despite this, traditional risk assessment tools underestimate true risk in this population.[3,4] Because of this as well as a variety of disease-specific factors that are discussed here, these patients are often undertreated in terms of prevention of cardiovascular disease.[5,6]

In this article, the authors summarize selected chronic inflammatory disorders and their associated cardiovascular disease risks. They discuss the use of nontraditional cardiac risk calculators and subclinical atherosclerosis imaging to aid in assessing cardiac risk. They also provide evidence-based treatment options for these unique patient populations.

Department of Internal Medicine, Division of Cardiology, 2799 West Grand Boulevard, Detroit, MI 48202, USA
* Corresponding author.
E-mail address: CRussel6@hfhs.org
Twitter: @CardioRheum (C.R.)

Med Clin N Am 106 (2022) 349–363
https://doi.org/10.1016/j.mcna.2021.11.010
0025-7125/22/© 2021 Elsevier Inc. All rights reserved.

Cardiac Manifestations of Inflammatory Disorders				
Vascular	Valvular	Pericardial	Myocardial	Conduction
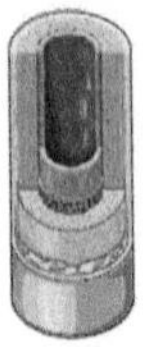	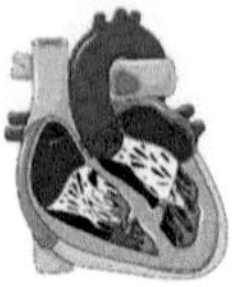	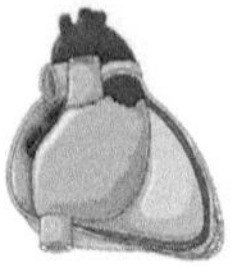	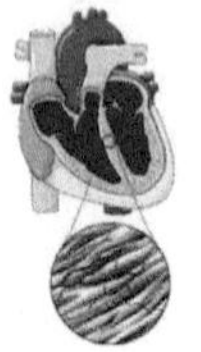	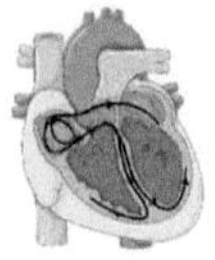
Atherosclerosis Vasculitis Thrombosis	Valvular Regurgitation Libman-Sacks Endocarditis	Pericarditis Pericardial Effusion	Hypertrophy Diastolic Dysfunction Fibrosis	Ventricular Arrhythmia AV block Supraventricular Tachycardia

Fig. 1. Cardiac manifestation of chronic inflammatory conditions and their clinical presentation. Images adapted with permission from www.smart.servier.com.

MECHANISM OF ATHEROSCLEROSIS IN INFLAMMATION

Systemic inflammation, mediated by both the innate and the adaptive immune system, contributes to cardiovascular disease through multiple mechanisms. Increased levels of activated neutrophils, reactive oxygen species, and proinflammatory cytokines lead to endothelial dysfunction, atherosclerosis, and thrombosis. Many of the proinflammatory cytokines, including tumor necrosis factor (TNF), interleukin-6 (IL-6), and IL-1, are present in chronic inflammatory diseases. They increase the risk of coronary artery disease by causing atherosclerosis, plaque instability, and plaque rupture.[1,2] Inflammation-induced microvascular dysfunction can also lead to stiffness and hypertrophy of cardiomyocytes, which may progress to diastolic dysfunction (**Fig. 2**). Myocardial infarction associated with inflammatory disease can cause systolic dysfunction.[7,8]

COMMONALITIES IN PATIENTS WITH INFLAMMATORY DISEASE

Although inflammatory diseases have different patterns of pathophysiology, risk, and symptoms, there are several commonalities in their care that are important in the prevention of cardiovascular disease. These include the following:

- Underrecognition of associated cardiovascular risk
- Inadequate cardiovascular risk screening
- Failure of traditional risk assessments
- Undertreatment of risk factors

Underrecognition of Associated Cardiovascular Risk

There is a lack of awareness of the association between inflammation and cardiovascular disease, on the part of both patients and clinicians. Only one-third of patients with rheumatoid arthritis (RA) are aware that their disease is associated with an increased risk of cardiovascular disease. Even more concerning, those at the highest

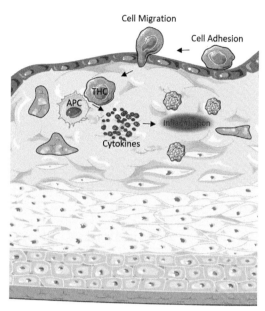

Fig. 2. Atherosclerotic plaque formation owing to inflammation. T-helper cells (THC) activated by antigen-presenting cells (APC) adhere to and migrate into the endothelial wall. This leads to production of various cytokines, contributing to vessel wall inflammation. In turn, lipids and lipoproteins are taken up by macrophages, dendritic cells, and smooth muscle cells to form lipid-laden foam cells. Images adapted with permission from www.smart. servier.com.

actual risk had the lowest perceived risk.[9] Although nearly all rheumatologists and infectious disease subspecialists are aware of the increased risk of cardiac disease in this patient population, awareness is only around 50% in primary care providers.[10]

Inadequate Cardiovascular Risk Screening

Patients with inflammatory diseases have a lower rate of screening for traditional cardiovascular risk factors than the general population, including routine lipid testing, diabetic screening, and screening for tobacco abuse.[5,11] In one study of 2035 patients affected with human immunodeficiency virus (HIV), only 19% of patients discussed cardiovascular disease with their providers, and only 31% discussed hypertension, hypercholesterolemia, family history of cardiovascular disease, or smoking.[11]

One reason for the lack of screening may be that many patients see their subspecialists (rheumatologist or infectious disease) as often as or more frequently than they see their primary care providers. This can complicate preventive care for several reasons. Subspecialty visits are spent focusing on a specific and often complicated disease process, leaving inadequate time for broader health discussions. Subspecialists may not have the same comfort with preventive screening tools or medication initiation, such as statins or diabetic medications, as primary care providers.[12,13] Furthermore, these clinical settings do not have the same resources as a primary care clinic, such as dedicated staff to perform routine blood pressure and diabetic medication titrations. In either clinic setting, there are additional barriers, including time constraints, insufficient visit frequency, and the competing demands of acute medical problems with preventive care.[5]

Failure of traditional risk assessments

Even when clinicians and patients align to address cardiovascular disease risk, traditional risk assessment tools significantly underestimate cardiovascular risk in patients with underlying inflammatory disorders.[3,4,14] In a retrospective study of 296 patients with systemic lupus erythematosus (SLE), the risk of myocardial infarction was discovered to be 10.1 times greater than that estimated using Framingham study risk factors. They were 17.0 times more likely than estimated to die of a cardiovascular cause and 7.9 times more likely to suffer a stroke.[4] A similar pattern of underestimation of cardiac risk with the use of traditional cardiac risk assessment tools is seen in all inflammatory conditions.

Many organizations, including the European League Against Rheumatism (EULAR) and the American Heart Association (AHA), suggest multiplying the traditional risk score by a correction factor to adjust for this underestimation. For example, they suggest multiplying calculated risk by 1.5 for RA and up to 2 in HIV.[15] This correction allows for a better estimation of cardiac risk in these patients and can lead to earlier initiation of appropriate preventive testing and medication initiation.

Undertreatment of risk factors

Despite several guidelines for cardiovascular disease risk management, implementation of appropriate preventive therapies in clinical practice remains suboptimal.[6,14,16] One reason for undertreatment of hyperlipidemia in particular is the overestimated perceived risk of statin-associated myalgias on the part of both clinicians and patients, many of whom already suffer from chronic pain.[17]

INFLAMMATORY DISEASES AND SPECIFIC CARDIOVASCULAR DISEASE RISK/MORBIDITY/MORTALITY

Although all chronic inflammatory diseases have increased cardiovascular disease risk, the following will be discussed in more detail:

- Rheumatoid arthritis
- Systemic lupus erythematosus
- Ankylosing spondylitis
- Psoriatic arthritis
- Gout
- Human immunodeficiency virus
- Inflammatory bowel disease (IBD)

RHEUMATOID ARTHRITIS

RA is the most common autoimmune arthritis, affecting approximately 1% of the population. There is a 3:1 female-to-male predominance, and the age of onset is typically between 30 and 60 years.[18] Compared with the general population, patients with RA have up to a 3 times higher risk of cardiovascular disease (**Table 1**), similar to the risk

Table 1	
Risk of selected disease with rheumatoid arthritis compared to the general population	
Diagnosis	**Relative Risk to General Population**
Cerebrovascular incident	1.48 (confidence interval [CI] 0.7–3.12)[23]
Myocardial infarction	2.00 (CI 1.23–3.29)[23]
Congestive heart failure	1.7 (CI 1.3–2.1)[24]

of diabetes.[19] Life expectancy can be shortened by 10 to 15 years, and up to 40% of deaths are attributable to cardiovascular causes.[20–22]

Comorbid Conditions

In addition to chronic inflammation, patients with RA have a higher prevalence of traditional cardiovascular risk factors, including hyperlipidemia, diabetes, hypertension, sedentary lifestyle, and obesity. An estimated one-third of patients with RA use tobacco products. The use of tobacco has been shown to promote arthritis disease activity and decrease response to antirheumatic therapy. They also have higher rates of depression and nonadherence, thought partially owing to disease-associated chronic pain. It was previously thought that these risk factors alone explained their cardiovascular disease risk; however, when compared with matched non-RA patients, their risk remains significantly higher.[23]

Many of the commonly prescribed therapies for RA carry a risk of cardiotoxicity. Chronic and high-dose corticosteroid use has been independently associated with increased risk of cardiovascular disease.[25] Similarly, use of nonsteroidal anti-inflammatory drugs, including cyclooxygenase inhibitors, used to treat joint pain is associated with 2 times increased cardiovascular risk. These medications can counteract the antiplatelet effects of aspirin and increases risk of coronary artery disease and heart failure.[26] Conversely, disease-modifying antirheumatic drugs, such as methotrexate, hydroxychloroquine, sulfasalazine, and leflunomide, effectively treat inflammation and pain while decreasing cardiovascular events in a dose-dependent relationship.[27] TNF-alpha inhibitors, although contraindicated in patients with heart failure, may normalize platelet reactivity, improve insulin resistance, and reduce subclinical atherosclerosis.[28]

Hyperlipidemia

Low-density lipoprotein (LDL) cholesterol is not always a reliable risk predictor in patients with active RA. In a phenomenon termed the "lipid paradox," inflammation in active disease is associated with lower levels of LDL cholesterol but increased cardiovascular risk. With initiation of treatment and resultant reduced disease activity, LDL levels increase and cardiovascular disease risk decreases. With treatment of inflammation, LDL-associated risk again tracks with the general population.[29,30]

Statin therapy has significant benefit in patients with RA, not only in the prevention of cardiovascular disease but also in the treatment of underlying inflammation itself. In patients with active disease who are initiated on statin therapy, levels of C-reactive protein (CRP), erythrocyte sedimentation rate, and proinflammatory cytokines (TNF, IL-1, IL-6) decrease. Reported disease activity, joint pain, and swelling also decreased.[31–33] Despite this, patients with RA are underscreened and undertreated for hyperlipidemia.[6,16]

SYSTEMIC LUPUS ERYTHEMATOSUS

SLE is a systemic autoimmune disease with multiorgan involvement. It more commonly affects African American women and women of child-bearing age.[34] As with other underlying inflammatory disorders, these patients are predisposed to inflammation-related endothelial dysfunction and accelerated atherosclerosis. The risk of coronary artery disease and myocardial infarction is 9 times higher in SLE patients than the general population and as much as 50 times higher than matched women without SLE.[35,36] SLE-specific autoantibodies can cause damage to the myocardium and cardiac valves, pericardial inflammation, and, in those with antiphospholipid antibodies, an increased risk of thrombotic events.[37,38] Cardiovascular disease is the leading cause of death in SLE.[39] Similar to the other inflammatory disorders, traditional risk scores significantly underestimate risk.[4]

ANKYLOSING SPONDYLITIS

Ankylosing spondylitis, strongly correlated to the presence of HLA-B23 surface antigen, is a systemic inflammatory disorder that typically manifests in the spine and sacroiliac joints. It is most commonly seen in young, white, male patients.[40] The most commonly associated cardiovascular manifestations include aortic root dilatation and calcification, aortic insufficiency, and conduction abnormalities. Aortic insufficiency is present in up to 20% of patients, and routine echocardiography at the time of presentation may be considered.[41] Patients also have an increased risk of atherosclerosis that is underestimated by most traditional risk scores. The exception is the Reynold's Risk Score, which includes CRP as a variable, and predicts risk with fair accuracy.[42,43] The use of subclinical atherosclerosis imaging, such as carotid intima medial thickness (CIMT), has been shown to improve the accuracy of risk assessment.[43,44]

PSORIATIC ARTHRITIS

Psoriatic arthritis, typically but not always accompanied by cutaneous psoriasis, carries an increased risk of myocardial infarction, peripheral vascular disease, and heart failure.[45] Inflammation in this disease accounts for 20% to 30% of the risk of acute myocardial infarction, and there are ongoing studies comparing various immunosuppression regimens with regression of coronary and carotid plaque burden.[46,47]

GOUT

Gout is a crystal-induced inflammatory joint disease typically associated with hyperuricemia. It affects approximately 1% of the population. Although patients with gout have a higher burden of traditional cardiovascular risk factors, gout has been shown to be an independent risk factor for cardiovascular mortality.[48] Ten percent of patients with gout will develop congestive heart failure versus 2% in the general population, and there appears to be a linear relationship between the risk of heart failure and serum urate concentrations.[49,50]

HUMAN IMMUNODEFICIENCY VIRUS

Advances in highly active antiretroviral therapy have dramatically improved the life expectancy of patients with HIV. As this population is living longer, cardiovascular disease has emerged as one of the major causes of non-AIDS–related mortality.[51] In addition to increased risk of both subclinical atherosclerosis and coronary artery disease, patients with HIV are susceptible to myocarditis and left ventricular dysfunction owing to viral and infiltrative cardiomyopathy.[52]

Newer antiretroviral therapy can have favorable effects not only in HIV-specific factors but also on cardiovascular risk factors. Treatment with antiretroviral therapy improves lipids and decreases systemic inflammation.[14,53] Unfortunately, some older regimens can cause weight gain, impaired left ventricular systolic function, and altered glucose and lipid metabolism. These are more often used in resource-poor settings where access to the newer drugs is limited.[14]

For treatment of hyperlipidemia, clinicians should be knowledgeable of the drug-drug interactions between statins and HIV therapy. Clinical pharmacists used in many HIV clinics can be especially helpful in these discussions. Because of these interactions, many patients with HIV will be unable to achieve goal LDL on statin monotherapy. For these patients, treatment with PCSK9 inhibitors have been shown to be an effective and safe option in HIV.[54]

INFLAMMATORY BOWEL DISEASE

IBD, including Crohn disease and ulcerative colitis, is an inflammatory disorder that predominantly affect the intestines. These disorders can also cause systemic inflammation, and up to 14% of patients will also have arthritis symptoms. IBD has an increased risk of venous thromboembolism. There is an increased risk of myocardial infarction and stroke in IBD, especially in younger patients and in women.[55,56] Fortunately, despite the increased cardiovascular event rates, death from cardiovascular disease has not been reliably shown to increase in IBD.[57]

PROPOSED TREATMENT APPROACHES FOR PRIMARY AND SECONDARY PREVENTION

With the development of new guidelines that include inflammation as a risk factor, there is hope that awareness of increased cardiovascular disease risk will continue to increase. The authors propose the following resources and additions to clinic practice:

- Guidelines and disease-specific risk calculators
- Multidisciplinary teams
- Imaging to improve risk assessment

Guidelines and Disease-specific Risk Calculators

There are now several guidelines acknowledging increased risk in chronic inflammatory conditions and HIV. EULAR provides recommendations for cardiovascular disease prevention in individual rheumatic and inflammatory musculoskeletal conditions.[58] The 2018 American College of Cardiology/AHA Cholesterol Guidelines include chronic inflammatory diseases and HIV as risk-enhancing factors to consider when treating hyperlipidemia.[59] There are also several disease-specific risk scores that have been or are being developed to address the inadequacy of traditional risk assessments (**Table 2**).

Multidisciplinary Care Teams

Intuitively, multidisciplinary teams in inflammatory conditions improve preventive screening and treatment.[10,12] There is an emerging field of Cardio-Rheumatology,

Table 2 Suggested disease-specific cardiac risk calculators	
Rheumatoid arthritis	• Expanded Cardiovascular Risk Prediction Score in Rheumatoid Arthritis[25] • QRISK3 (includes RA as an additional risk factor as well as chronic steroid use) • Multiply traditional risk score by 1.5[58]
Systemic lupus erythematosus	• QRISK3 (includes SLE as an additional risk factor)
Ankylosing spondylitis	• Reynolds Risk Score (includes CRP)[42]
Human immunodeficiency virus	• Multiply traditional risk score by 2[14]

similar to Cardio-Oncology,[60] in which specialists from both fields work closely together to provide optimal lifestyle and medication regimens with the goal of decreasing risk. Across the country, there is also growing support for joint Cardio-Rheum clinics, where patients are seen by their rheumatologist as well as a cardiologist focused on preventive cardiovascular health. This is important in both primary and secondary prevention of cardiovascular events.

IMAGING TO IMPROVE RISK ASSESSMENT

Given the unreliability of traditional risk assessment models, there is growing support for subclinical atherosclerosis imaging to help guide preventive strategies, including carotid intima-media thickness (CIMT) and coronary artery calcium scoring.

Carotid Intima-Media Thickness

One of the best validated atherosclerosis imaging techniques for patients with inflammatory conditions is the ultrasound CIMT measurement. By measuring the thickness between the carotid intima and media, this noninvasive imaging modality detects carotid atherosclerotic vascular disease in its early stages before the development of symptoms or adverse events (**Fig. 3**). This can be especially useful in patients with underlying inflammatory disorders, where risk is uncertain (**Table 3**).

Further demonstrating the relationship between inflammation and atherosclerosis, treatment of the underlying inflammation in the diseases described above can aid in regression of CIMT.[61,66] This can help clinicians monitor disease activity as well as lower cardiovascular disease risk.

Coronary Artery Calcium Scoring

Patients with inflammatory disorders have a higher prevalence and severity of coronary artery calcium owing to an atherogenic effect of chronic systemic inflammation.[67]

Table 3
Carotid intima-media thickness in specific inflammatory disorders

Rheumatoid arthritis	Threefold increase (44% vs 15%) in carotid atherosclerosis compared with non-RA patients with similar risk profiles[61]
Systemic lupus erythematosus	Higher CIMT and presence of carotid plaque are predictive of cardiovascular events, including stroke, myocardial infarction, and need for coronary revascularization[62]
Human immunodeficiency virus	CIMT is increased in HIV-related risk factors, such as viral load and absence of antiretroviral therapy[63] Patients with HIV are shown to have a higher CIMT than non-HIV patients at the same age[64] Increased CIMT is associated with a higher mortality[53]
Psoriatic arthritis	The addition of CIMT to traditional risk assessment, such as Systematic Coronary Risk Evaluation (SCORE), resulted in upgrade and reclassification of risk to very high risk in 1/3 of patients[65]
Ankylosing spondylitis	CIMT is increased significantly compared with healthy controls[44]
Inflammatory bowel disease	CIMT increases proportionate to disease activity. In patients with higher CRP levels, CIMT increased similarly to patients with RA[58]

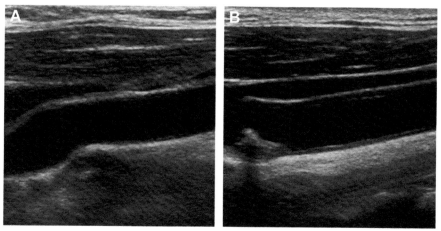

Fig. 3. (*A*) Normal carotid artery ultrasound with normal CIMT. (*B*) Thickened CIMT with atherosclerotic plaque visualized on the left. Images provided by Dr. Karthikeyan Ananthasubramaniam, Director of Carotid Ultrasound Laboratory at Henry Ford Hospital.

The use of Coronary Artery Calcium Scoring can detect coronary artery disease before the development of symptomatic and obstructive coronary disease. In particular, it can be helpful when either patients or clinicians are uncertain of whether to start lipid-lowering therapy, and both US and European guidelines support its use for this purpose[68] (**Fig. 4**).

Echocardiography to detect subclinical heart failure

Echocardiographic strain imaging, similar to its use in chemotherapy monitoring, can predict subclinical myocardial dysfunction in inflammatory disease, including RA and SLE. This can help clinicians initiate or adjust therapy before the development of irreversible dysfunction.[69,70]

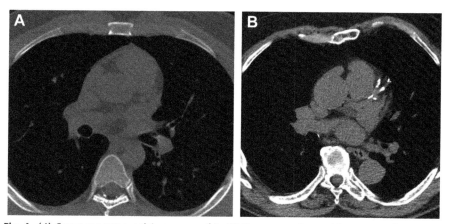

Fig. 4. (*A*) Coronary artery calcium score of 0. (*B*) Coronary artery calcium score of 1776 in a patient with RA, with severe calcifications in the left anterior descending and its branching diagonal arteries.

SECONDARY PREVENTION

Inflammation is an important factor in secondary prevention of myocardial infarction. In the CANTOS (Canakinumab Anti-Inflammatory Thrombosis Outcomes Study) trial, patients with an elevated level of high-sensitivity CRP postmyocardial infarction had lower incidence of recurrent cardiovascular events when treated with canakinumab, a monoclonal antibody targeting IL-1β.[71] Although this trial excluded patients with chronic inflammatory and immunosuppressed states, it serves as an important proof of concept that inflammation is independently associated with risk of recurrent myocardial infarction even when other traditional treatments, including lipid lowering therapy, remain constant.

Recent data have suggested that low-dose colchicine has a role for secondary prevention through anti-inflammatory mechanism in coronary artery disease. Colchicine at a dose of 0.5 mg daily reduces inflammatory response and lowers the risk of ischemic cardiovascular events both in patients with a recent acute coronary event and in those with stable chronic coronary artery disease.[72]

Patients with inflammatory disorders have an increased risk of recurrent events.[58] In patients with underlying inflammatory disorders, communication and coordination of care between cardiology and other providers become even more vital in reducing risk of recurrence. These patients should be aggressively treated for their underlying inflammation as well as for their traditional risk factors.

SUMMARY

Inflammation plays a well-established role in the development and progression of atherosclerosis and contributes to endothelial dysfunction and thrombosis. Patients exposed to chronic inflammation are at an increased risk of cardiovascular disease, including coronary artery disease, stroke, and heart failure independent of associated traditional cardiac risk factors.

Providing adequate preventive cardiac care for patients with underlying inflammatory conditions offers a unique set of challenges for the clinician. Traditional risk assessment models significantly and consistently underestimate their risk of cardiovascular events. This leads to missed opportunities for prevention. The use of additional imaging and laboratory testing can play an important additional role in their risk assessment. Given the multisystem nature of inflammatory disorders, coordination between all providers is uniquely important in screening and treatment of underlying risk.

CLINICS CARE POINTS

- Individuals exposed to chronic inflammation are at an increased risk of developing cardiovascular disease, including coronary artery disease, stroke, and heart failure.
- Traditional risk assessment tools and calculators (Framingham Risk Score, Atherosclerotic Cardiovascular Disease (ASCVD) calculator, and so forth) underestimate the true cardiac risk in these patients.
- The use of imaging (carotid intima media thickness, coronary calcium scoring, echocardiography) and laboratory testing (high-sensitivity C-reactive protein, erythrocyte sedimentation rate) aid in the assessment of risk and can be used to help guide preventive care and timing of medication initiation.

- Collaborative care between cardiology, rheumatology, infectious disease and primary care providers allows for more accurate risk assessment and improved treatment of risk.

DISCLOSURE

The authors have nothing to disclose.

REFERENCES

1. Hansson GK. Inflammation, atherosclerosis, and coronary artery disease. N Engl J Med 2005;352(16):1685–95.
2. Libby P, Ridker PM, Hansson GK, Leducq Transatlantic Network on A. Inflammation in atherosclerosis: from pathophysiology to practice. J Am Coll Cardiol 2009; 54(23):2129–38.
3. Alemao E, Cawston H, Bourhis F, et al. Comparison of cardiovascular risk algorithms in patients with vs without rheumatoid arthritis and the role of C-reactive protein in predicting cardiovascular outcomes in rheumatoid arthritis. Rheumatology (Oxford) 2017;56(5):777–86.
4. Esdaile JM, Abrahamowicz M, Grodzicky T, et al. Traditional Framingham risk factors fail to fully account for accelerated atherosclerosis in systemic lupus erythematosus. Arthritis Rheum 2001;44(10):2331–7.
5. Bartels CM, Kind AJ, Everett C, et al. Low frequency of primary lipid screening among Medicare patients with rheumatoid arthritis. Arthritis Rheum 2011;63(5): 1221–30.
6. Toms TE, Panoulas VF, Douglas KM, et al. Statin use in rheumatoid arthritis in relation to actual cardiovascular risk: evidence for substantial undertreatment of lipid-associated cardiovascular risk? Ann Rheum Dis 2010;69(4):683–8.
7. Westermann D, Lindner D, Kasner M, et al. Cardiac inflammation contributes to changes in the extracellular matrix in patients with heart failure and normal ejection fraction. Circ Heart Fail 2011;4(1):44–52.
8. Paulus WJ, Tschope C. A novel paradigm for heart failure with preserved ejection fraction: comorbidities drive myocardial dysfunction and remodeling through coronary microvascular endothelial inflammation. J Am Coll Cardiol 2013;62(4): 263–71.
9. Ghosh-Swaby OR, Kuriya B. Awareness and perceived risk of cardiovascular disease among individuals living with rheumatoid arthritis is low: results of a systematic literature review. Arthritis Res Ther 2019;21(1):33.
10. Bartels CM, Roberts TJ, Hansen KE, et al. Rheumatologist and primary care management of cardiovascular disease risk in rheumatoid arthritis: patient and provider perspectives. Arthritis Care Res (Hoboken) 2016;68(4):415–23.
11. Sherer R, Solomon S, Schechter M, et al. HIV provider-patient communication regarding cardiovascular risk: results from the AIDS Treatment for Life International Survey. J Int Assoc Provid AIDS Care 2014;13(4):342–5.
12. Lakshmi S, Beekmann SE, Polgreen PM, et al. HIV primary care by the infectious disease physician in the United States - extending the continuum of care. AIDS Care 2018;30(5):569–77.
13. Fultz SL, Goulet JL, Weissman S, et al. Differences between infectious diseases-certified physicians and general medicine-certified physicians in the level of comfort with providing primary care to patients. Clin Infect Dis 2005;41(5): 738–43.

14. So-Armah K, Benjamin LA, Bloomfield GS, et al. HIV and cardiovascular disease. Lancet HIV 2020;7(4):e279–93.

15. Ryom L, Boesecke C, Bracchi M, et al. Highlights of the 2017 European AIDS Clinical Society (EACS) Guidelines for the treatment of adult HIV-positive persons version 9.0. HIV Med 2018;19(5):309–15.

16. van Breukelen-van der Stoep DF, van Zeben D, Klop B, et al. Marked underdiagnosis and undertreatment of hypertension and hypercholesterolaemia in rheumatoid arthritis. Rheumatology (Oxford) 2016;55(7):1210–6.

17. Nissen SE. Statin denial: an internet-driven cult with deadly consequences. Ann Intern Med 2017;167(4):281–2.

18. van der Woude D, van der Helm-van Mil AHM. Update on the epidemiology, risk factors, and disease outcomes of rheumatoid arthritis. Best Pract Res Clin Rheumatol 2018;32(2):174–87.

19. Lindhardsen J, Ahlehoff O, Gislason GH, et al. The risk of myocardial infarction in rheumatoid arthritis and diabetes mellitus: a Danish nationwide cohort study. Ann Rheum Dis 2011;70(6):929–34.

20. Avina-Zubieta JA, Thomas J, Sadatsafavi M, et al. Risk of incident cardiovascular events in patients with rheumatoid arthritis: a meta-analysis of observational studies. Ann Rheum Dis 2012;71(9):1524–9.

21. Kitas GD, Gabriel SE. Cardiovascular disease in rheumatoid arthritis: state of the art and future perspectives. Ann Rheum Dis 2011;70(1):8–14.

22. Naz SM, Symmons DP. Mortality in established rheumatoid arthritis. Best Pract Res Clin Rheumatol 2007;21(5):871–83.

23. Solomon DH, Karlson EW, Rimm EB, et al. Cardiovascular morbidity and mortality in women diagnosed with rheumatoid arthritis. Circulation 2003;107(9):1303–7.

24. Maradit-Kremers H, Nicola PJ, Crowson CS, et al. Cardiovascular death in rheumatoid arthritis: a population-based study. Arthritis Rheum 2005;52(3):722–32.

25. Solomon DH, Greenberg J, Curtis JR, et al. Derivation and internal validation of an expanded cardiovascular risk prediction score for rheumatoid arthritis: a Consortium of Rheumatology Researchers of North America Registry Study. Arthritis Rheumatol 2015;67(8):1995–2003.

26. Nissen SE, Yeomans ND, Solomon DH, et al. Cardiovascular safety of celecoxib, naproxen, or ibuprofen for arthritis. N Engl J Med 2016;375(26):2519–29.

27. Choi HK, Hernan MA, Seeger JD, et al. Methotrexate and mortality in patients with rheumatoid arthritis: a prospective study. Lancet 2002;359(9313):1173–7.

28. Di Minno MN, Ambrosino P, Peluso R, et al. Lipid profile changes in patients with rheumatic diseases receiving a treatment with TNF-alpha blockers: a meta-analysis of prospective studies. Ann Med 2014;46(2):73–83.

29. Robertson J, Peters MJ, McInnes IB, et al. Changes in lipid levels with inflammation and therapy in RA: a maturing paradigm. Nat Rev Rheumatol 2013;9(9):513–23.

30. Myasoedova E, Crowson CS, Kremers HM, et al. Lipid paradox in rheumatoid arthritis: the impact of serum lipid measures and systemic inflammation on the risk of cardiovascular disease. Ann Rheum Dis 2011;70(3):482–7.

31. McCarey DW, McInnes IB, Madhok R, et al. Trial of Atorvastatin in Rheumatoid Arthritis (TARA): double-blind, randomised placebo-controlled trial. Lancet 2004;363(9426):2015–21.

32. Maki-Petaja KM, Booth AD, Hall FC, et al. Ezetimibe and simvastatin reduce inflammation, disease activity, and aortic stiffness and improve endothelial function in rheumatoid arthritis. J Am Coll Cardiol 2007;50(9):852–8.

33. Lv S, Liu Y, Zou Z, et al. The impact of statins therapy on disease activity and inflammatory factor in patients with rheumatoid arthritis: a meta-analysis. Clin Exp Rheumatol 2015;33(1):69–76.

34. Jain D, Halushka MK. Cardiac pathology of systemic lupus erythematosus. J Clin Pathol 2009;62(7):584–92.

35. Jonsson H, Nived O, Sturfelt G. Outcome in systemic lupus erythematosus: a prospective study of patients from a defined population. Medicine (Baltimore) 1989; 68(3):141–50.

36. Manzi S, Meilahn EN, Rairie JE, et al. Age-specific incidence rates of myocardial infarction and angina in women with systemic lupus erythematosus: comparison with the Framingham Study. Am J Epidemiol 1997;145(5):408–15.

37. Tincani A, Rebaioli CB, Taglietti M, et al. Heart involvement in systemic lupus erythematosus, anti-phospholipid syndrome and neonatal lupus. Rheumatology (Oxford) 2006;45(Suppl 4):iv8–13.

38. Moyssakis I, Tektonidou MG, Vasilliou VA, et al. Libman-Sacks endocarditis in systemic lupus erythematosus: prevalence, associations, and evolution. Am J Med 2007;120(7):636–42.

39. Knight JS, Kaplan MJ. Cardiovascular disease in lupus: insights and updates. Curr Opin Rheumatol 2013;25(5):597–605.

40. Taurog JD, Chhabra A, Colbert RA. Ankylosing spondylitis and axial spondyloarthritis. N Engl J Med 2016;375(13):1303.

41. Klingberg E, Svealv BG, Tang MS, et al. Aortic regurgitation is common in ankylosing spondylitis: time for routine echocardiography evaluation? Am J Med 2015; 128(11):1244–12450.e1.

42. Navarini L, Caso F, Costa L, et al. Cardiovascular risk prediction in ankylosing spondylitis: from traditional scores to machine learning assessment. Rheumatol Ther 2020;7(4):867–82.

43. Rueda-Gotor J, Genre F, Corrales A, et al. Relative risk chart score for the assessment of the cardiovascular risk in young patients with ankylosing spondylitis. Int J Rheumatol 2018;2018:1847894.

44. Yuan Y, Yang J, Zhang X, et al. Carotid intima-media thickness in patients with ankylosing spondylitis: a systematic review and updated meta-analysis. J Atheroscler Thromb 2019;26(3):260–71.

45. Ahlehoff O, Gislason GH, Charlot M, et al. Psoriasis is associated with clinically significant cardiovascular risk: a Danish nationwide cohort study. J Intern Med 2011;270(2):147–57.

46. Eder L, Dey A, Joshi AA, et al. Cardiovascular diseases in psoriasis and psoriatic arthritis. J Rheumatol Suppl 2019;95:20–7.

47. Di Minno MN, Iervolino S, Peluso R, et al. Carotid intima-media thickness in psoriatic arthritis: differences between tumor necrosis factor-alpha blockers and traditional disease-modifying antirheumatic drugs. Arterioscler Thromb Vasc Biol 2011;31(3):705–12.

48. Lottmann K, Chen X, Schadlich PK. Association between gout and all-cause as well as cardiovascular mortality: a systematic review. Curr Rheumatol Rep 2012;14(2):195–203.

49. Huang H, Huang B, Li Y, et al. Uric acid and risk of heart failure: a systematic review and meta-analysis. Eur J Heart Fail 2014;16(1):15–24.

50. Krishnan E. Gout and the risk for incident heart failure and systolic dysfunction. BMJ Open 2012;2(1):e000282.
51. Miller CJ, Baker JV, Bormann AM, et al. Adjudicated morbidity and mortality outcomes by age among individuals with HIV infection on suppressive antiretroviral therapy. PLoS One 2014;9(4):e95061.
52. Barbaro G. HIV-associated cardiomyopathy etiopathogenesis and clinical aspects. Herz 2005;30(6):486–92.
53. Mangili A, Polak JF, Quach LA, et al. Markers of atherosclerosis and inflammation and mortality in patients with HIV infection. Atherosclerosis 2011;214(2):468–73.
54. Adhyaru BB, Jacobson TA. Role of non-statins, LDL-C thresholds, and special population considerations: a look at the updated 2016 ACC Consensus Committee Recommendations. Curr Atheroscler Rep 2017;19(6):29.
55. Feng W, Chen G, Cai D, et al. Inflammatory bowel disease and risk of ischemic heart disease: an updated meta-analysis of cohort studies. J Am Heart Assoc 2017;6(8):e005892.
56. Card TR, Zittan E, Nguyen GC, et al. Disease activity in inflammatory bowel disease is associated with arterial vascular disease. Inflamm Bowel Dis 2021;27(5): 629–38.
57. Sun HH, Tian F. Inflammatory bowel disease and cardiovascular disease incidence and mortality: a meta-analysis. Eur J Prev Cardiol 2018;25(15):1623–31.
58. Agca R, Heslinga SC, Rollefstad S, et al. EULAR recommendations for cardiovascular disease risk management in patients with rheumatoid arthritis and other forms of inflammatory joint disorders: 2015/2016 update. Ann Rheum Dis 2017; 76(1):17–28.
59. Grundy SM, Stone NJ, Bailey AL, et al. 2018 AHA/ACC/AACVPR/AAPA/ABC/ ACPM/ADA/AGS/APhA/ASPC/NLA/PCNA Guideline on the Management of Blood Cholesterol: a report of the American College of Cardiology/American Heart Association Task Force on Clinical Practice Guidelines. Circulation 2019;139(25): e1082–143.
60. Yoo BW. Embarking on a career in cardio-rheumatology. J Am Coll Cardiol 2020; 75(12):1488–92.
61. Ristic GG, Lepic T, Glisic B, et al. Rheumatoid arthritis is an independent risk factor for increased carotid intima-media thickness: impact of anti-inflammatory treatment. Rheumatology (Oxford) 2010;49(6):1076–81.
62. Kao AH, Lertratanakul A, Elliott JR, et al. Relation of carotid intima-media thickness and plaque with incident cardiovascular events in women with systemic lupus erythematosus. Am J Cardiol 2013;112(7):1025–32.
63. Kaplan RC, Sinclair E, Landay AL, et al. T cell activation and senescence predict subclinical carotid artery disease in HIV-infected women. J Infect Dis 2011; 203(4):452–63.
64. Krikke M, Arends JE, Van Lelyveld S, et al. Greater carotid intima media thickness at a younger age in HIV-infected patients compared with reference values for an uninfected cohort. HIV Med 2017;18(4):275–83.
65. Martinez-Vidal MP, Andres M, Jovani V, et al. Role of carotid ultrasound and systematic coronary risk evaluation charts for the cardiovascular risk stratification of patients with psoriatic arthritis. J Rheumatol 2020;47(5):682–9.
66. Roman MJ, Moeller E, Davis A, et al. Preclinical carotid atherosclerosis in patients with rheumatoid arthritis. Ann Intern Med 2006;144(4):249–56.
67. Giles JT, Szklo M, Post W, et al. Coronary arterial calcification in rheumatoid arthritis: comparison with the multi-ethnic study of atherosclerosis. Arthritis Res Ther 2009;11(2):R36.

68. Orringer CE, Blaha MJ, Blankstein R, et al. The National Lipid Association scientific statement on coronary artery calcium scoring to guide preventive strategies for ASCVD risk reduction. J Clin Lipidol 2021;15(1):33–60.

69. Fine NM, Crowson CS, Lin G, et al. Evaluation of myocardial function in patients with rheumatoid arthritis using strain imaging by speckle-tracking echocardiography. Ann Rheum Dis 2014;73(10):1833–9.

70. Buss SJ, Wolf D, Korosoglou G, et al. Myocardial left ventricular dysfunction in patients with systemic lupus erythematosus: new insights from tissue Doppler and strain imaging. J Rheumatol 2010;37(1):79–86.

71. Ridker PM, Everett BM, Thuren T, et al. Antiinflammatory therapy with canakinumab for atherosclerotic disease. N Engl J Med 2017;377(12):1119–31.

72. Tardif JC, Kouz S, Waters DD, et al. Efficacy and safety of low-dose colchicine after myocardial infarction. N Engl J Med 2019;381(26):2497–505.

Women's Cardiovascular Health
Selecting the Best Contraception

Monika Sanghavi, MD[a],*, Jourdan E. Triebwasser, MD, MA[b]

KEYWORDS

- Cardiovascular disease • Pregnancy • Contraception • Cardio-obstetrics

KEY POINTS

- Contraception counseling needs to be part of the cardiovascular visit for women with significant cardiovascular morbidity, at high risk of cardiovascular complications during pregnancy, or on cardiac medications that are teratogenic.
- Estrogen-based contraception should be avoided in women at high risk of thromboembolic events, multiple or uncontrolled cardiovascular risk factors, or at risk of heart failure with fluid retention.
- Use of references such as the US Medical Eligibility Criteria for Contraception can help clinicians appropriately counsel women on contraception.

INTRODUCTION

The scope of cardiovascular (CV) care for woman has expanded over the past several years. This expanded scope is due to better understanding of CV risk in women, the growing concern for maternal CV morbidity and mortality during pregnancy, and acknowledgment of the cardiologist's role in education when prescribing teratogenic medications. Effective contraception is essential, especially in those with contraindications for pregnancy. Effective contraception allows for optimal timing of pregnancy and discontinuation of teratogenic cardiac medications before conception.

Traditionally, contraception counseling has been deferred to obstetrician-gynecologists (OBGyn) and primary care physicians; however, cardiologists may need to initiate the discussion to ensure patients receive timely and comprehensive care. Basic understanding of contraceptives and implications in specific cardiovascular diseases will allow partnership with primary care and OBGyn colleagues.[1]

[a] Division of Cardiology, University of Pennsylvania, 3400 Civic Center Boulevard, Philadelphia, PA 19104, USA; [b] Division of Maternal-Fetal Medicine, University of Michigan, 1500 East Medical Center Drive, Ann Arbor, MI 48109, USA
* Corresponding author.
E-mail address: Monika.Sanghavi@pennmedicine.upenn.edu
Twitter: @MonSangh (M.S.); @JourdieTMD (J.E.T.)

Med Clin N Am 106 (2022) 365–376
https://doi.org/10.1016/j.mcna.2021.11.011
0025-7125/22/Published by Elsevier Inc.

The goal of this review is to provide cardiologists a concise summary of the types of contraception based on efficacy, contraception considerations in specific cardiovascular conditions, and resources for clinicians.

HORMONAL CHANGES DURING THE MENSTRUAL CYCLE

The menstrual cycle is a coordinated hormonal cycle that results in the release of a mature oocyte (ovulation). The cyclic changes in anterior pituitary hormones (luteinizing hormone [LH] and follicle stimulating hormone [FSH]) and gonadal hormones (estrogen and progesterone) are shown later (**Fig. 1**). The average menstrual cycles last 21 to 35 days[2] and is divided into follicular and luteal phases. The follicular phase begins with menses ("period"). The duration of menstrual bleeding averages 5 days but can be as long as 7 days. The LH surge triggers ovulation.

The luteal phase begins with ovulation and lasts approximately 14 days. The ovarian follicle cells remaining after ovulation become the corpus luteum, which produces progesterone. If a pregnancy does not occur, the corpus luteum degenerates, leading to a drop in progesterone and the next menstrual cycle. Several forms of contraception inhibit ovulation including the combined hormonal contraceptives (CHC), which include an estrogen and progestin.

TYPES OF CONTRACEPTION BY EFFICACY

Without contraception, it is anticipated that 85 of 100 women would become pregnant in 1 year. Thus, all of the following forms of contraception reduce that risk. However, there are methods that are significantly more effective than others (**Fig. 2**). The efficacy of contraceptive methods demonstrated in clinical trials may vary significantly from the clinical effectiveness.[3] Effectiveness highly depends on correct and consistent use.

Sterilization

Both male and female sterilization are safe and effective methods of contraception. Women who do not desire future pregnancy are candidates for sterilization, which can be accomplished by laparoscopy, at the time of cesarean delivery, or by minilaparotomy. Women interested in sterilization should be counseled on risk of failure, risk of regret, and effective alternatives.[4] Compared with female sterilization,

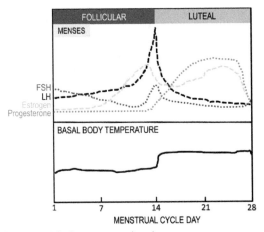

Fig. 1. Hormonal changes with the menstrual cycle.

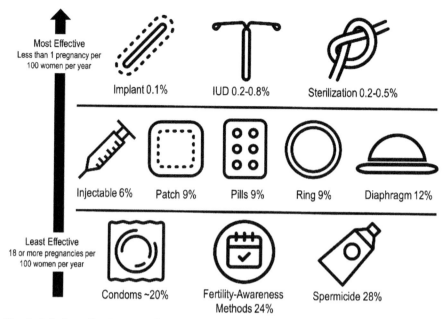

Fig. 2. Relative effectiveness of various forms on contraception, modified from the CDC "Effectiveness of Family Planning Methods". IUD, intrauterine device.

vasectomy is more effective, safer, and less expensive. Vasectomy should be considered for couples interested in permanent contraception, particularly for women with increased surgical risk related to cardiovascular disease.

Long-Acting Reversible Contraceptive Methods

Long-acting reversible contraceptive methods (LARC) methods include the etonogestrel contraceptive implant and intrauterine devices (IUD). There are several types of hormonal IUD that contain levonorgestrel. A nonhormonal copper IUD is also available. The primary benefit of LARC methods is that they are highly effective and have high user satisfaction.[5,6] In addition, two-thirds of women who select an LARC method are still using that method 3 years later, versus approximately one-third of non-LARC users.[7] Some considerations and noncontraceptive benefits of various LARC methods are shown in **Table 1**.

The primary mechanism of action for the etonogestrel implant is suppression of ovulation.[8] Whereas, ovulation is suppressed in a minority of women using the levonorgestrel IUDs. The primary mechanism of action for these devices is change in amount and viscosity of cervical mucus that inhibits sperm migration. The copper IUD prevents pregnancy by inhibiting sperm viability and migration. IUDs are not associated with increased risk of increased hypertension (HTN), stroke, venous thromboembolism (VTE), fluid retention, or QT prolongation in trials.[9]

Injectable Contraceptives

Depot medroxyprogesterone acetate (DMPA) is the only injectable contraceptive available in the United States. It is given intramuscularly or subcutaneously every 3 months. DMPA is often used for menstrual suppression in women who cannot tolerate estrogen or do not desire LARC methods.[10] Weight gain is commonly

Table 1
Characteristics of verious long-acting reversible contraceptive methods

LARC Method	FDA-Approved Duration	Considerations
Etonogestrel implant	3 y	• Generally, lightens menstrual bleeding • Some women experience unscheduled spotting or irregular bleeding • Not associated with increased risk of increased HTN, HL, MI, stroke, VTE, or fluid retention in trials[9]
Copper IUD	10 y	• Avoidance of exogenous hormones • Continuation of pre-IUD bleeding pattern. Bleeding may be heavier or more painful, especially in first cycles after placement. • Can be used for emergency contraception • Not associated with increased risk of increased HTN, stroke, VTE, fluid retention, or QT prolongation in trials[9]
Levonorgestrel (LNG) IUD	—	• Reduces menstrual bleeding or may cause amenorrhea (no menstrual bleeding) • Reduces painful periods • Reduces risk of endometrial and ovarian cancer • Not associated with increased risk of increased HTN, stroke, VTE, fluid retention, or QT prolongation in trials[9]
52 mg LNG IUD (commercial names Mirena, Liletta)	6 y	• Most likely to cause amenorrhea (20% at 1 y, 30%–50% at 3 y)
19.5 mg LNG IUD (commercial name Kyleena)	5 y	—
13.5 mg LNG IUD (commercial name Skyla)	3 y	• Least likely to cause amenorrhea

reported with DMPA, but average weight gain is limited and may not differ from other hormonal forms of contraception.[11] DMPA may worsen bone loss because it induces a hypoestrogenic state; this could potentiate the possible bone loss associated with long-term warfarin therapy.[10] There are some studies that suggest VTE risk is increased, although evidence of this is weak. Long-term DMPA has been shown to induce unfavorable changes in lipid profiles such as increase in total cholesterol, triglycerides, and low-density lipoprotein and reduction in high-density lipoprotein.[9]

Combined Hormonal Contraceptives

CHC include a combination of estrogen (various dosages) and progestins (4 different generations). Progestin differs from progesterone in that it is synthetically derived. Except drospirenone (fourth generation), progestins do not have mineralocorticoid properties that endogenous progesterone has. Modern CHC use significantly lower doses of estrogen than early oral contraceptive pills (OCPs). CHC methods include OCPs, patches, and rings. CHC effectiveness is limited by frequency of administration—daily for pills, weekly for the patch, and monthly to annually for ring contraceptives. CHCs are often selected due to noncontraceptive benefits, which may include reduction in heavy or irregular menstrual bleeding, dysmenorrhea, acne, and hirsutism. The primary risk associated with CHC is a small increased risk of venous and arterial thrombosis, although for most populations the absolute risk is low. The relative risk of myocardial infarction from arterial thrombosis is 1.40 to 1.8 for low (20 μg) to medium (30–40 μg) dose estrogen preparations.[9] There is a 2- to 4-fold increased risk of VTE, which may be influenced by both the estrogen and progestin components. Third and fourth generation progestins are associated with higher VTE risk than second-generation progestins.[9]

Estrogen and progestins can affect the QT interval. Estrogen lengthens the QT interval. The effect of progestins on the QT interval varies based on the progestin generation and the androgenic potential. The first- to third-generation progestins shorten the QT, whereas fourth-generation progestins have been shown to lengthen the QT interval.[12] The change in QT duration is minimal, 4 ms, and registry data suggest no difference in cardiac events.[13]

There is no significant weight change for patients on combined hormonal. The risk of hypertension is discussed separately in this article.

Progestin-Only Pill

The progestin-only pill is a daily medication with typical use effectiveness similar to CHC without many of the concerns associated with estrogen. However, progestin-only pills must be taken at the same time daily to be effective. Noncontraceptive benefits include decreased menstrual bleeding and reduction in dysmenorrhea. Norethindrone POPs, the formulation available in the United States, are not associated with blood pressure elevations, increased risk of VTE, fluid retention, changes in lipid profile, or QTc prolongation.

Barrier Methods

Barrier methods include male and female condoms, cervical caps, and diaphragms; these can be used with or without spermicide. Condoms are readily available and provide protection from many sexually transmitted infections. Cervical caps and diaphragms have to be fitted, which limits availability.

Fertility Awareness-Based Methods

Fertility awareness-based methods rely on physiologic changes of normal, ovulatory menstrual cycles, and the functional viability of sperm and ova. These methods avoid hormone exposure, but require regular cycles, the ability to track changes, and a supportive partner to avoid intercourse during fertile windows.

CLINICIAN RESOURCES FOR CHOOSING CONTRACEPTION

The World Health Organization (WHO) created a document with medical eligibility criteria for contraception for global guidance.[14] The fifth edition was published in 2015. Based on the recommendations from the WHO, the Center for Disease Control (CDC) has adapted the guidelines for use in the United States, US Medical Eligibility Criteria for Contraceptive Use (USMEC), and has committed to keeping the recommendations up to date based on critical appraisal of the literature. The last iteration of the recommendations came out in 2016. The recommendations are available to the clinician in many easy-to-use formats including a summary chart, an eligibility criteria wheel, and an app available on most mobile devices.[15] These guidelines can be used when consulting with patients regarding their contraceptive options.

The American College of Obstetricians and Gynecologists has published a practice bulletin[16] and an expert option paper[10] to help fill some of the gaps that are not addressed within the CDC guidelines for women with coexisting medical and cardiac conditions, respectively.

The US MEC guidelines are based on a 4-category system and whether contraception is being initiated (I) or continued (C).

- *Category 1*: condition for which there is no restriction for the use of the contraceptive method.
- *Category 2*: condition for which the advantages generally outweigh the theoretic/proven risks.
- *Category 3*: condition for which the theoretic or proven risks usually outweigh the advantages.
- *Category 4*: condition that represents an unacceptable health risk of the contraceptive method.

CONTRACEPTION CONSIDERATIONS IN HIGH-RISK WOMEN

Counseling on contraception needs to involve shared decision-making. Factors that should be considered are effectiveness, method-related risks, noncontraceptive benefits, individual preferences, and risk of unplanned pregnancy. From a cardiologist's viewpoint, the most important considerations are contraception efficacy and avoidance of cardiovascular risk.

Hypertension

High-dose OCPs with at least 50 μg estrogen and 1 to 4 mg progestin can cause hypertension in 5% of users.[4] Although CHC formulations have changed significantly since their introduction in the 1960s with marked reduction in hormonal content, blood pressure elevations have been reported even in normotensive women with lower doses of estrogen (30 μg).[5]

Mechanism of induced hypertension is not completely understood, but is partially due to stimulation of hepatic synthesis of angiotensin by estrogen, which ultimately leads to an increase in aldosterone levels and hence sodium and water retention.[17]

Influence of oral contraceptive on risk of hypertension differs in women according to ethnicity, family history of hypertension, obesity, and age.

Higher susceptibility to incident hypertension is reported in those with a family history of hypertension and those of black race. A prospective study of oral contraceptive and hypertension demonstrated that older women are more likely to develop hypertension than younger women, and long-term users (>6 years) were more likely to develop HTN.[18] A history of hypertension in pregnancy may also increase the risk of hypertension with oral contraceptives.[19]

More significant blood pressure changes are seen with older generation OCP likely due to the higher doses of estrogen. Progestin dose may also play a role in risk of blood pressure elevation. Monophasic versus biphasic or triphasic formulations have increased risk of hypertension. However, POP seem NOT to be associated with hypertension.[18]

In one small prospective trial evaluating oral OCP versus the barrier method, the average blood pressure increase after 3 years in the OCP group was 9.2 mm Hg in systolic blood pressure (SBP) and 5 mm Hg in diastolic blood pressure (DBP), and BP increased further after 4 years.[20] The delta blood pressure may be smaller with newer contraceptives.[21] Fortunately, blood pressure changes with CHC are reversible. Blood pressure returns to pretreatment levels usually within 4 weeks and almost always within 3 months after CHC is discontinued. In hypertensive women, a decrease in SBP of up to 15 mm Hg has been observed after discontinuation of OCPs.[22]

Oral contraceptives with the newer generation progestin, drospirenone, with antimineralocorticoid properties lower SBP when combined with estrogen.

Treatment of CHC-induced HTN is discontinuation. Even when well controlled, women with hypertension are not advised to take CHC, as the risk is thought to outweigh the benefit. All other forms of contraception can be considered. When SBP is greater than or equal to 160 mm Hg or DBP greater than or equal to 100 mm Hg or there is evidence of vascular disease, CHC is contraindicated (**Box 1**) and DMPA is avoided.

USMEC recommendations for patients with hypertension are based on the premise that no other risk factors for cardiovascular disease are present. When multiple risk factors exist, CHC may increase a patient's cardiovascular risk to an unacceptable level and should not be used (see **Box 1**). Clinical judgment is advised by USMEC (category 2) when using CHC in women with history of gestational hypertension due to a relative increased risk of myocardial infarction and VTE.

A proposed algorithm for contraception selection in patients with hypertension was recently published in JAMA. Although not clinically validated, it may help provide guidance to the busy clinician.[17]

Other Cardiovascular Risk Factors

Contraceptive considerations for other cardiovascular risk factors are listed in **Table 2**.

These considerations are based on USMEC guidelines and expert opinion. When multiple cardiovascular risk factors are present or single-risk factors such as hypertension or hyperlipidemia are not controlled, CHC is not recommended.[23]

CONTRACEPTION IN WOMEN WITH UNDERLYING CARDIOVASCULAR DISEASE
Congenital Heart Disease

Overall CHC is considered safe in simple congenital heart disease (CHD) such as secundum atrial septal defect, patent foramen ovale, and small ventricular septal

---

Box 1
Contraindications[a] to combined hormonal contraception (based on World Health Organization and Centers of Disease Control recommendations)[27]

Age ≥35 years and smoking ≥15 cigarettes per day

≥ 2 risk factors for arterial cardiovascular disease (older age, smoking, DM, HTN, low HDL, high LDL, or TG)

HTN (SBP ≥160 mm Hg or DBP ≥100 mm Hg)

Venous thromboembolism

Known ischemic heart disease

History of stroke

Complicated valvular heart disease (pulmonary hypertension, atrial fibrillation, bacterial endocarditis)

[a] USMEC Category 4. A condition that represents an unacceptable health risk if the contraceptive method is used.

Abbreviations: DM, diabetes mellitus; HDL, high density lipoprotein; HTN, hypertension; LDL, low density lipoprotein; SBP, systolic blood pressure; TG, triglycerides.

Table 2
Contraceptive considerations in women with elevated cardiovascular risk[23,27]

Hypertension	In women with hypertension, even if well controlled → avoid CHC. In women with severely uncontrolled hypertension with SBP ≥160 or DBP ≥100, CHC is contraindicated.
Dyslipidemia	LDL-C >160 mg/dL or multiple cardiac risk factors → consider alternate nonhormonal contraceptive methods such as IUD[a,b]
Diabetes	Diabetes type I or II, <35 y of age, duration <20 y, no other risk factors, absence of micro- or macrovascular disease → CHC may be considered Otherwise, progestin-only or IUD may be considered. DMPA should be avoided if DM >20 y or underlying vascular disease
Smoking	Smoking >15 cigarettes/d and ≥35 y of age →alternative contraceptive methods such as IUD, POC
Obesity	BMI >30 kg/m² → COC can be considered weighing risks and benefits or alternate contraceptive method such as IUD or POC
Age	Healthy, nonsmoking women, ok to continue oral contraceptive until age 40 y and possibly until menopause weighing risks and benefits.

Abbreviations: BMI, body mass index; COC, combined oral contraceptives; DM, diabetes mellitus; HTN, hypertension; LDL-C, low density lipoprotein cholesterol; POC, progestin-only contraceptives.
  [a] Theoretic concern about effect on lipids with levonorgestrel IUD.
  [b] Certain progestin-only contraception may increase the risk of thrombosis, although this increase is substantially less than with COCs. The effects of DMPA might persist for some time after discontinuation.
Adapted from Shufelt and Bairey Merz. Contraceptive Hormone Use and Cardiovascular Disease.

defects. They are also considered safe in aortic coarctation, aortic stenosis, and repaired tetralogy of fallot. However, there is concern that CHC are harmful for women with congenital heart disease who are at increased risk of thromboembolic events, specifically cyanotic disease, Fontan physiology, D-transposition, single ventricle physiology, and pulmonary arterial hypertension.[10]

LARC methods may be particulary beneficial for women with congenital heart disease with unique considerations regarding type. Pain and cervical manipulation during insertion and removal of an IUD can elicit a vagal reaction in as many as 5% of women. It is potentially dangerous in those with pulmonary HTN or Fontan repair. Therefore, insertion and removal of IUDs in these women should be performed with appropriate cardiovascular monitoring for hypotension and arrhythmias, anesthesia support, and adequate pain relief.[10] Because of concerns associated with IUD implantation, subdermal implants may be a preferred option due to ease of insertion. There have been case reports of infective endocarditis with IUD insertion[24]; however, the American Heart Association and the American College of Gynecology recommend against routine antibiotic prophylaxis for IUD insertion or removal.[10,25]

Dilated Cardiomyopathy/Peripartum Cardiomyopathy/Cardiac Transplant

In patients with dilated cardiomyopathy and a depressed ejection fraction, pregnancy can result in significant morbidity for the mother and fetus.[26] In addition, the goal-directed medical therapy has potential fetal toxicity. Similarly, patients with peripartum cardiomyopathy have a significant risk associated with future pregnancies that highly depends on left ventricular (LV) function recovery. Those who do not recover their LV function have a significant mortality risk associated with future pregnancies,[26] and reliable contraception is an important part of the medical regimen.

USMEC guidelines specifically address contraception in peripartum cardiomyopathy, and recommendations are influenced by LV function. CHCs are not recommended due to the theoretic risk of fluid retention and or arrhythmias, whereas POP, IUD, and DMPA are all considered safe (category 1 and 2). Among the acceptable contraception options, the relative efficacy of each needs to be considered against the risk of unintended pregnancy, especially in those with severe LV dysfunction.

Dilated cardiomyopathy and other forms of cardiomyopathies are not independently addressed in the USMEC guidelines; however, the recommendations for peripartum cardiomyopathy are extrapolated.[26]

Pregnancy in women with prior heart transplant is feasible but considered high risk. Avoidance of pregnancy for at least 1 to 2 years posttransplant is recommended due to the high risk of rejection during this time[9]; therefore, contraception considerations are critical.

USMEC has general recommendations for solid organ transplants that are based on whether the transplant was complicated or uncomplicated. Contraception counseling in cardiac transplant patients should include USMEC recommendations for solid organ transplants AND any other cardiovascular comorbidities that are present.

In the uncomplicated transplant patient without comorbidities, all forms of contraception are allowable including CHC (category 2). However, because of the high rate of comorbidities in this population, IUDs are often the preferred agent.[9]

Complicated transplants are defined as those that show evidence of graft failure, rejection, or transplant vasculopathy. In this population, there are several restrictions on contraceptives. CHC are contraindicated (category 4). De novo IUD insertion is not recommended due to the concern for increased risk of infection in the setting of immunosuppression (category 3). However, continuation of an existing device is considered safe (category 2). Progesterone-only contraception is permissible. However, DPMA is not recommended in patients with dyslipidemia or evidence of bone loss.

Valvular Heart Disease

Valvular diseases are divided into uncomplicated valvular disease and complicated valvular disease. Women with uncomplicated disease may use any form of contraception. Complicated valvular heart disease, defined by coexisting atrial fibrillation, pulmonary hypertension, or prior endocarditis,[27] is thought to have an increased risk for thrombosis. CHC is not recommended (category 4), whereas POPs, LARC, barrier method, and DMPA are all considered safe for use (category 1). Although barrier methods are considered safe, the lower efficacy rate needs to be weighed against the risk associated with contraception failure and risk of pregnancy.

Arrhythmias/Systemic Anticoagulation

Women on systemic anticoagulation present a unique concern. Direct oral anticoagulants are not recommended during pregnancy and need to be discontinued. Warfarin has dose-dependent adverse fetal effects that make unplanned pregnancy undesirable. DMPA injection has not been found to carry additional risk of hematoma formation in the setting of systemic anticoagulation. LARC methods are generally considered good options. The copper IUD is associated with heavier menstrual bleeding, which may pose a concern for patients already on anticoagulation, thus levonorgestrel IUD may be better tolerated.[9]

Women at risk of ventricular arrhythmias (long QT syndrome, hypertrophic cardiomyopathy, ischemic cardiomyopathy, severely reduced LV systolic function) have a theoretic risk from exposure to contraceptive agents that prolong the QT interval. However, the theoretic risk has not translated to clinical risk,[9] and there is no evidence

Table 3
Summary of contraceptive recommendations for women with cardiovascular conditions

Anticoagulation[16]	All progestin-only methods are acceptable for women taking anticoagulants Copper IUD may increase bleeding, whereas levonorgestrel IUD significantly reduces blood loss and is an excellent option
History of Stroke or MI[27]	CHC is contraindicated. DMPA is not recommended. If event occurred while on therapy such as POP, implant, or LNG-IUD, continuation may not be recommended. Copper-IUD can be used; however, bleeding risk needs to be considered
POTS[10]	CHC can cause fluid retention, which may relieve symptoms with POTS
Congenital Heart Disease[10]	Depends on the type of CHD. For simple CHD, all forms of contraception are acceptable. For those with cyanotic or more complex CHD, CHC are avoided. IUD placement with caution due vagal reaction
Cardiac Transplant[9]	Recommendations depend on whether or not transplant is complicated (see discussion). Also, higher efficacy contraception should be considered in the first 1–2 y due to higher risk of rejection
Peripartum Cardiomyopathy[27]	CHC should be avoided if possible; most other forms of contraception can be considered.
Valvular Heart Disease[27]	Recommendations depends on whether it is complicated or uncomplicated (see discussion). CHC contraindicated in complicated VHD. Progestin-only methods are considered safe in both

Abbreviations: CHD, congenital heart disease; MI, myocardial infarction; POTS, postural orthostatic tachycardia syndrome; VHD, valvular heart disease.

that contraception of any kind triggers the occurrence of arrhythmias. Therefore, those with isolated arrhythmias (ventricular extra beats, atrioventruclar nodal tachycardia, isolated supraventricular tachycardia, or ventricular tachycardia in long-QT syndrome), CHC can likely be used[28] but is not specifically addressed in the USMEC recommendations.

However, in atrial fibrillation CHC are not recommended due to elevated risk of thromboembolism.[28] There is paucity of data on whether the increased thrombogenic risk of CHC is counterbalanced by therapeutic anticoagulation; therefore, it should be avoided even on those who are fully anticoagulated.

Additional Cardiovascular Diseases

Current recommendations for additional cardiovascular disease are summarized in **Table 3**.

SUMMARY

Choosing a particular contraceptive method is a highly individualized decision; each woman should retain autonomy and the ability to choose a method that is compatible with her personal values, level of comfort, reproductive desires, and underlying medical issues. There are both nonhormonal and hormonal forms of pregnancy prevention and each comes with its unique risk and benefit profile. Methods differ in terms of effectiveness, side-effect profile, drug interactions, use of hormones, cost, confidentiality concerns, and the degree of control women have over their use.

Contraception counseling is an important part of the comprehensive care of women with cardiovascular disease, and it is important for cardiologists to be able to initiate the discussion and contribute to the decision-making process for optimal care of these patients.

CLINICS CARE POINTS

- Estrogen-based contraception (even low dose) can elevate blood pressure. Discontinuation of CHC is the first step in management of CHC-related hypertension. Even if blood pressure is well controlled, CHC should be avoided.
- Estrogen-based contraception should be avoided in women at high risk of thromboembolic events, multiple or uncontrolled cardiovascular risk factors, or at risk of heart failure with fluid retention.
- Use of references such as the USMEC can help clinicians appropriately counsel women on contraception.

DISCLOSURE

The authors have nothing to disclose.

REFERENCES

1. Lindley KJ, Bairey Merz CN, Davis MB, et al. Contraception and Reproductive Planning for Women With Cardiovascular Disease: JACC Focus Seminar 5/5. J Am Coll Cardiol 2021;77(14):1823–34.
2. Committee on Practice Bulletins—Gynecology. Practice bulletin no. 128: diagnosis of abnormal uterine bleeding in reproductive-aged women. Obstet Gynecol 2012;120(1):197–206.
3. Trussell J. Contraceptive failure in the United States. Contraception 2011;83(5): 397–404.
4. American College of Obstetricians and Gynecologists' Committee on Practice Bulletins—Gynecology. ACOG Practice Bulletin No. 208: Benefits and Risks of Sterilization. Obstet Gynecol 2019;133(3):e194–207.
5. Peipert JF, Zhao Q, Allsworth JE, et al. Continuation and satisfaction of reversible contraception. Obstet Gynecol 2011;117(5):1105–13.
6. Moray KV, Chaurasia H, Sachin O, et al. A systematic review on clinical effectiveness, side-effect profile and meta-analysis on continuation rate of etonogestrel contraceptive implant. Reprod Health 2021;18(1):4.
7. Diedrich JT, Zhao Q, Madden T, et al. Three-year continuation of reversible contraception. Am J Obstet Gynecol 2015;213(5):662.e1-8.
8. Committee on Practice Bulletins-Gynecology. Long-Acting Reversible Contraception Work Group. Practice Bulletin No. 186: Long-Acting Reversible Contraception: Implants and Intrauterine Devices. Obstet Gynecol 2017;130(5):e251–69.
9. Maroo A, Chahine J. Contraceptive Strategies in Women With Heart Failure or With Cardiac Transplantation. Curr Heart Fail Rep 2018;15(3):161–70.

10. Gynecologic Considerations for Adolescents and Young Women With Cardiac Conditions: ACOG Committee Opinion, Number 813. Obstet Gynecol 2020; 136(5):e90–9.

11. Lopez LM, Ramesh S, Chen M, et al. Progestin-only contraceptives: effects on weight. Cochrane Database Syst Rev 2016;8:CD008815.

12. Sedlak T, Shufelt C, Iribarren C, et al. Oral contraceptive use and the ECG: evidence of an adverse QT effect on corrected QT interval. Ann Noninvasive Electrocardiol 2013;18(4):389–98.

13. Abu-Zeitone A, Peterson DR, Polonsky B, et al. Oral contraceptive use and the risk of cardiac events in patients with long QT syndrome. Heart Rhythm 2014; 11(7):1170–5.

14. Gaffield ML, Kiarie J. WHO medical eligibility criteria update. Contraception 2016;94(3):193–4.

15. US Medical Eligibility Criteria (US MEC) for Contraceptive Use, 2016 | CDC. Published November 19, 2020. Available at: https://www.cdc.gov/reproductivehealth/contraception/mmwr/mec/summary.html. Accessed April 24, 2021.

16. ACOG Practice Bulletin No. 206: Use of Hormonal Contraception in Women With Coexisting Medical Conditions. Obstet Gynecol 2019;133(2):e128–50.

17. Shufelt C, LeVee A. Hormonal Contraception in Women With Hypertension. JAMA 2020. https://doi.org/10.1001/jama.2020.11935.

18. Chasan-Taber L, Willett WC, Manson JE, et al. Prospective study of oral contraceptives and hypertension among women in the United States. Circulation 1996;94(3):483–9.

19. Khaw KT, Peart WS. Blood pressure and contraceptive use. Br Med J (Clin Res Ed) 1982;285(6339):403–7.

20. Weir RJ, Briggs E, Mack A, et al. Blood pressure in women taking oral contraceptives. Br Med J 1974;1(5907):533–5.

21. Wilson ES, Cruickshank J, McMaster M, et al. A prospective controlled study of the effect on blood pressure of contraceptive preparations containing different types and dosages of progestogen. Br J Obstet Gynaecol 1984;91(12):1254–60.

22. Lubianca JN, Moreira LB, Gus M, et al. Stopping oral contraceptives: an effective blood pressure-lowering intervention in women with hypertension. J Hum Hypertens 2005;19(6):451–5.

23. Shufelt CL, Bairey Merz CN. Contraceptive hormone use and cardiovascular disease. J Am Coll Cardiol 2009;53(3):221–31.

24. Meyerowitz EA, Prager S, Stout K, et al. Endocarditis following IUD insertion in a patient with tetralogy of Fallot. BMJ Case Rep 2019;12(2). https://doi.org/10.1136/bcr-2018-227962.

25. Wilson W, Taubert KA, Gewitz M, et al. Prevention of infective endocarditis: guidelines from the American Heart Association: a guideline from the American Heart Association Rheumatic Fever, Endocarditis, and Kawasaki Disease Committee, Council on Cardiovascular Disease in the Young, and the Council on Clinical Cardiology, Council on Cardiovascular Surgery and Anesthesia, and the Quality of Care and Outcomes Research Interdisciplinary Working Group. Circulation 2007;116(15):1736–54.

26. Sedlak T, Merz CNB, Shufelt C, et al. Contraception in Patients with Heart Failure. Circulation 2012;126(11):1396–400.

27. Curtis KM, Tepper NK, Jatlaoui TC, et al. U.S. Medical Eligibility Criteria for Contraceptive Use, 2016. MMWR Recomm Rep 2016;65(3):1–103.

28. Roos-Hesselink JW, Cornette J, Sliwa K, et al. Contraception and cardiovascular disease. Eur Heart J 2015;36(27):1728–34.

Noninvasive Imaging for the Asymptomatic Patient
How to Use Imaging to Guide Treatment Goals?

Juliette Kathleen Logan, MD*, Michael Parker Ayers, MD*

KEYWORDS

- Subclinical atherosclerosis • Cardiac prevention • Coronary artery calcium scan
- Coronary computed tomography angiography • Carotid intima-media thickness
- Ankle-brachial index • Toe-brachial index

KEY POINTS

- Subclinical atherosclerosis imaging identifies individuals at higher risk of cardiovascular disease before events occur so that preventative measures can be taken.
- The main methods of subclinical atherosclerosis imaging are coronary artery calcium scan, coronary computer tomography angiography, carotid intima-medial thickness, ankle-brachial index, and toe-brachial index.
- This review explores recent studies and discuss guidelines on each of these imaging modalities.

INTRODUCTION

Atherosclerosis precedes the development of clinical cardiovascular disease (atherosclerotic cardiovascular disease [ASCVD]), including myocardial infarction, cerebrovascular accident, and limb ischemia. Subclinical atherosclerosis refers to the existence of atherosclerotic lesions before an individual's first major cardiovascular symptom or event. Atherosclerosis has numerous stages, from fatty streaks to atheromas to fibroatheromas to complex plaques. Through this evolution, atherosclerosis is generally a disease with a long "incubation" period. Subclinical atherosclerosis can first be detected in North Americans during their second and third decades of life, but cardiovascular events usually occur after several decades of disease progression.[1] Despite the relatively indolent time course, complications such as myocardial infarction, acute limb ischemia, and stroke typically occur suddenly. By intervening early on the right patient, preventative medications should be able to reduce the

Division of Cardiovascular Medicine, University of Virginia, Heart and Vascular Center Fontaine, 500 Ray C. Hunt Drive, Charlottesville, VA 22903, USA
* Corresponding authors.
E-mail addresses: jkl9cv@hscmail.mcc.virginia.edu (J.K.L.); mpa2h@hscmail.mcc.virginia.edu (M.P.A.)

Med Clin N Am 106 (2022) 377–388
https://doi.org/10.1016/j.mcna.2021.11.012
0025-7125/22/© 2021 Elsevier Inc. All rights reserved.

complications of progressive atherosclerosis. Despite the long incubation time, many patients are not on any preventative medications at the time of their first event.

Identifying those who would benefit from early intervention, however, remains challenging. Current methods of assessing atherosclerosis risk such as ASCVD Framingham Risk Score and Pooled Cohort Equation have limited predictive value. These risk scores do not incorporate information about genetics or lifestyle, and are also less accurate in women, nonwhite populations, and in younger age groups. The PESA (Progression of Early Subclinical Atherosclerosis) study demonstrated that almost half of the asymptomatic individuals had subclinical atherosclerosis despite being considered low risk based on traditional risk factor models.[2] Analysis and quantification of subclinical atherosclerosis can assist in more accurately assessing risk where standard calculators fail.

Diagnosis of coronary artery disease (CAD) has traditionally relied on symptoms and functional tests of ischemia. Ischemic testing focuses on detection of flow-limiting coronary artery lesions and not on the detection of subclinical or nonobstructive atherosclerosis. Noninvasive imaging modalities, including coronary artery calcium (CAC) scan, coronary computer tomography angiography (CCTA), carotid intima-media thickness (CIMT), and the ankle-brachial index (ABI), allow for the detection of subclinical atherosclerosis, identifying those at risk before a clinically significant event occurs.

PHYSIOLOGY OF ATHEROSCLEROSIS

Unstable plaque progression is the sine qua non of acute vascular event. Roughly speaking, plaques are composed of 2 components: fibrous cap and necrotic lipid core.[3] Negative remodeling through the increasing size of the necrotic core and thinning of the fibrous cap predisposes to plaque rupture and acute vascular events. Plaque composition, rather than absolute plaque volume, is most closely related to risk of plaque rupture. The aim of subclinical atherosclerosis imaging is to identify atherosclerosis at the subclinical phase in order to assess an individual's risk of future event (**Fig. 1**). Subclinical atherosclerosis imaging assumes that the greater the burden of atherosclerosis, the greater the likelihood that unstable atherosclerosis will be present or develop in the future. Studies have shown that intensive treatment with statins reduces total plaque burden by decreasing necrotic core volume and increasing fibrous cap thickness, stabilizing plaques, and decreasing risk of plaque rupture.[4,5] Given lipid-lowering therapy's ability to halt plaque progression and evolution of high-risk plaque features, identifying those at elevated risk so they may initiate pharmacotherapy is of vital importance.[2]

CORONARY ARTERY CALCIUM SCORING

With iterative remodeling of the coronary vasculature due to dyslipidemia and inflammation, extracellular calcifications accumulate in the media. Spotty calcification or microcalcification coalesce over time by increasing in density within the intimal layer.[6] Coronary artery calcium scoring uses noncontrast CT in order to quantify the presence and extent of CAC within the epicardial vessels; this is done using the original protocol described to quantify CAC using CT by Agatston in 1990, which defines coronary calcium as a lesion greater than or equal to 1 mm^2 and greater than 130 Hounsfield units.[7] The calcium score is determined by the product of the calcified plaque area and maximal calcium lesion density (from 1 to 4 based on Hounsfield units), with the CAC score being the sum of these individual scores in each epicardial coronary artery. Standardized categories have been developed, with scores of 0 indicating the absence of calcified plaque, 1 to 10 minimal plaque, 11 to 100 mild plaque, 101 to

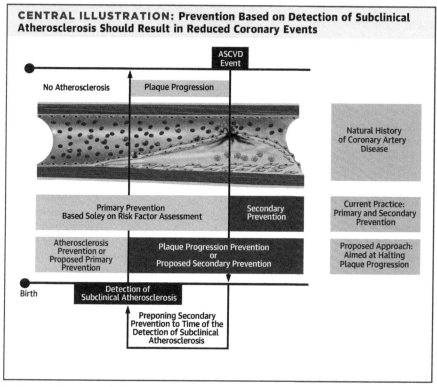

CENTRAL ILLUSTRATION: Prevention Based on Detection of Subclinical Atherosclerosis Should Result in Reduced Coronary Events

Fig. 1. The detection of subclinical atherosclerosis allows for the initiation of lipid-lowering therapy to halt plaque progression before an event occurs. (*From* Ahmadi, A. et al. with permission.)

400 moderate plaque, and greater than 400 severe plaque. From these calcium scores, a calcium percentile is generated by comparing the subject's score with others of the same age, sex, and ethnicity.[8] Higher than 75th percentile is considered high risk, irrespective of the score, and indicates premature atherosclerosis.

CAC scoring is best used for asymptomatic patients with borderline risk profiles, such as 2.5% to 7.5% 10-year risk of ASCVD events. For such asymptomatic patients, CAC can further risk stratify based on the presence of subclinical atherosclerosis to drive therapy. CAC scores are particularly likely to reclassify patients when they are 0 or greater than 100. A CAC score of 0 often reclassifies risk from borderline or intermediate to low. For those patients, subsequent focus should be placed on emphasizing beneficial dietary and lifestyle changes rather than pharmacotherapy. Analysis of the Multi-Ethnic Study of Atherosclerosis (MESA) data compared 13 negative risk markers and found that CAC 0 resulted in the greatest downward shift in risk estimation and in the largest net risk reclassification.[9] However, it should be noted that patients with higher risk subtypes as those with diabetes, active tobacco use, or family history of premature CAD may require pharmacotherapy despite a CAC score of 0. A CAC score greater than 100 often reclassifies risk from borderline to intermediate. For these patients, subsequent focus should include not just lifestyle but also strong consideration for lipid-lowering pharmacotherapy.[10] CAC can also be used for patient populations with ASCVD risks greater than 7.5%, particularly when there is a strong patient or provider desire to avoid lipid lower therapies. For example, a patient intolerant to statin therapy but with an ASCVD greater than 7.5% may be "de-risked" by a CAC score of 0. The minimum time interval for consideration of repeating a CAC scan in a primary prevention population with an initial CAC score of 0 is about 4 to 5 years. The rationale behind this interval is that after 5 years, 25% of patients with a CAC score of 0 will convert to a nonzero score.[6]

The MESA evaluated 6814 asymptomatic patients aged 45 to 84 years from different ethnic groups including Hispanic, Black, Chinese, and Caucasian cohorts.[11] This landmark paper discovered that the predictive power of CAC exists across all races included in the trial. The hazard ratio (HR) for any coronary event increased from 3.61 for a CAC score between 1 and 100 to an HR of 9.67 for a CAC score greater than 300. For each ethnic group within the MESA study, doubling of the CAC score increased the risk of a major coronary event by 15% to 35% and the risk of any coronary event by 18% to 39%.[12,13] Results from the MESA trial were incorporated in the MESA calculator, which allows providers to incorporate CAC score when calculating 10-year ASCVD risk.

The CAC Consortium examined sex differences in calcified plaque and found that the average age for detection of a CAC score greater than zero was 37 and 46 years of age for men and women, respectively.[14] Based on these findings, guidelines suggest CAC scores in men and women older than 40 and 50 years, respectively. In practice, CAC scores are typically obtained in men older than 35 years and women older than 45 years who have risk factors such as family history of cardiovascular disease. Given the natural progression of atherosclerosis formation, it becomes a lower yield test in much younger patients, as fatty streaks are not identifiable on CT due to the lack of associated calcifications.[6] In addition, the CAC Consortium found that across CAC subgroups, women had fewer calcified lesions, fewer calcified vessels, and a lower CAC volume compared with men of the same age. Interestingly, women within the same CAC score subgroup had fewer but larger sized calcified lesions (on average) when compared with their male counterparts.[14] These differences, likely driven by sex hormones, are important to highlight, as the clinical significance and relative risk of a 40-year-old woman who has any coronary calcium is worse than a 40-year-old man with the same CAC score. Likewise, when looking at the age of 50, a man who has a score of greater than 100 is at high risk, but a woman with a score of greater than 100 is a very high-risk patient.[6]

The incorporation of CAC scanning in guidelines has varied throughout the years, but their role in risk stratification has increased in most recent guidelines. Screening for Heart Attack Prevention and Education was the first guideline to incorporate CAC, although this was met with controversy.[15] The 2010 ACC/AHA Risk Assessment Guideline included CAC assessment as a class IIa recommendation, stating CAC was reasonable for risk assessment in asymptomatic adults at intermediate risk and for all diabetic patients older than 40 years.[16] In 2012, the European Society of Cardiology awarded a similar class IIa recommendation, suggesting CAC for CV risk assessment in asymptomatic adults at moderate risk.[17] The 2013 American College of Cardiology/American Heart Association (ACC/AHA) Cholesterol and Risk Guidelines created an entirely risk factor–based pooled cohort equation using the same risk factors as the 2010 version but with different weightings, now modified by race. CAC was downgraded to a class IIb recommendation specifically for those not in their 4 primary risk categories. The most recent update of ACC/AHA guidelines currently endorse the use of CT coronary calcium scoring to refine risk estimates in patients with risk between 5% and 20% over 10 years[10]; this is similarly indicated in the 2017 SCCT (Society of Cardiovascular Computer Tomography) indications recommending CAC for adult men and women with 10-year ASCVD risk of 5% to 20%. The SCCT guidelines extend the recommendation for those less than 5% 10-year risk if patients have another risk enhancing condition such as premature family history of coronary disease or inflammatory rheumatologic disease.[18]

The primary limitation of CAC scoring is radiation exposure. Requiring roughly 1 mSv, obtaining a CAC score is about 30% more radiation than annual background radiation from environmental exposure (0.7 mSv).[8] Initially expensive, CAC cost has declined steadily in cost to around $100 per scan. Advantages include high reproducibility and speed—taking only 10 to 15 minutes of scanner time with only a few seconds of acquisition time.[6] Unlike CCTA, heart rate control is not needed.

CORONARY COMPUTER TOMOGRAPHY ANGIOGRAPHY

CCTA is a noninvasive, contrast-enhanced study that can be used to detect coronary artery disease, characterize disease burden, and evaluate the degree of coronary stenosis.[19] During CCTA, patients receive iodinated contrast to visualize the coronary system, with image acquisition during an inspiratory breath hold. For optimal image acquisition, certain CT scanners require a lower target heart rate, ideally less than 60 beats per minute, for which β-blockers are often administered.[20]

CCTA is now most commonly used to assess primarily symptomatic patients. In current European Society of Cardiology (ESC) and National Institute for Health and Care Excellence guidelines, CCTA is preferred over stress testing for initial assessment of suspected coronary symptoms and in stable chest pain.[21] This clinical utility is driven by the strong ability of CCTA to not only effectively rule out obstructive CAD with high negative predictive value but also to diagnose nonobstructive disease. The SCOT-HEART (Computed Tomography Coronary Angiography for the Prevention of Myocardial Infarction) trial randomized patients with stable chest pain and suspected coronary disease to CCTA plus standard care with functional stress testing versus standard of care alone.[22,23] The CCTA plus standard care arm found an increase in the initiation of preventative therapies such as aspirin and statins for patients with increased atherosclerotic burden, with fewer prescriptions for those with less atherosclerotic burden. Five-year follow-up impressively found that primary endpoint of mortality from coronary artery disease or nonfatal myocardial infarction was lower (2.3%) in the CCTA arm compared with the standard care arm (3.9%). The earlier PROMISE (Prospective Multicenter Imaging Study for Evaluation of Chest Pain) trial demonstrated similar results in regard to the prognostic value and robust cardiovascular event prediction of CCTA compared with functional testing and standard care in the setting of stable chest pain.[24] Prognostic superiority of CCTA in PROMISE was even more pronounced in a subgroup analysis of patients with type 2 diabetes mellitus.[25] The benefits seen in SCOT-HEART and PROMISE are likely due to preventative medicine prescriptions for patients who needed them the most and derive the most benefit.

Yet, how much benefit do patients without chest pain receive from CCTA versus CAC alone? The CONFIRM registry was an international multicenter study of individuals who underwent CCTA and CAC scoring.[26] In analyses of subsets of patients without chest pain, the investigators evaluated the additive contribution of CCTA-defined risk assessment compared with the utilization of clinical risk factors with CAC. Both CAC and CCTA significantly improved performance of standard risk factor prediction models for all-cause mortality and the composite outcome. The incremental discriminatory value associated with their inclusion was most pronounced for the composite outcome. The C-statistic assessing the predictive power of tradition risk factors for the composite outcome was 0.71. For traditional risk factors plus the addition of CAC, the C-statistic was 0.75. Adding CCTA to risk factors plus CAC further improved the C-statistic to 0.77. Thus, CCTA does offer statistical improvement in risk prediction and reclassification for the composite endpoint of death and myocardial infarction compared with CAC alone. The modest improvement in the C-statistic from 0.75 to 0.77, however, begs the question if incremental benefit is worth the increase in cost, expertise, dye exposure, and radiation dose.

PARADIGM (Progression of Atherosclerotic Plaque Determined by Computed Tomographic Angiography Imaging) was a multinational observation registry composed of 2252 patients without known CAD who underwent serial CCTA at 2-year intervals.[27] On follow-up, patients on statins had slower atherosclerosis progression with more stabilization of plaques, including a significant reduction in plaque growth defined by annualized percent atheroma volume greater than the median of the study population (HR: 0.796; 95% confidence interval: 0.687–0.925; p = 0.003). A subsequent analysis of the same study demonstrated that statins were associated with a substantial reduction in number of high-risk plaque features and an increase in plaque calcifications, suggestive of plaque stabilization for patients taking statins. Just as CAC in asymptomatic populations directs preventative therapies based on plaque burden, these studies demonstrate the important role of CCTA in the symptomatic patient in defining the composition and stability of the underlying plaques.

Limitations for CCTA include low target heart rates for optimal image acquisition, the use of iodinated contrast injection that may be allergenic or nephrotoxic, and radiation exposure (roughly 2–5 mSv).[19] Advantages again include high reproducibility and additional, albeit modest, risk stratification compared with CAC alone.

CAROTID INTIMA-MEDIA THICKNESS

CIMT is the thickness of the intimal and medial layer of the carotid artery wall measured via ultrasound and is considered a marker for early atherosclerosis of all vascular beds, including the coronaries.[28] Using the epidemiologic Atherosclerosis Risk in Communities study population with a follow-up period of almost 15 years, the addition of CIMT and carotid plaque assessment to traditional cardiovascular risk prediction models reclassified 23% of study participants.[29] This reclassification was most profound in the intermediate risk group (5%–20% 10-year risk) where 61.9% of participants were reclassified as low risk with the addition of CIMT and carotid plaque assessment to their overall cardiovascular risk assessment. Notably, more study participants were reclassified to a lower risk group (12.4%) compared with participants reclassified to a higher risk group (10.8%) with the addition of CIMT and carotid plaque assessment.

A calculated IMT score incorporating measurements made at the common and internal carotid artery was calculated among the MESA cohort to calculate age, sex, and ethnicity matched percentiles added to cardiovascular risk assessment, which included the Framingham Risk Score and CAC score.[30] The net reclassification improvement (NRI) was 11.1% in a model using the Framingham Risk Score and a positive CAC score, whereas the NRI was 16.1% in a model combining the IMT score to a positive CAC score and Framingham Risk Score. This analysis noted that IMT can efficaciously predict coronary heart disease events when used alone, or it can provide incremental value when added to both the Framingham Risk Score and CAC score. Although CIMT provides incremental benefit when added to the CAC score for risk assessment, it likely should not be used in lieu of the CAC score in the appropriate age groups (men older than 40 years, woman older than 50 years), given robust data demonstrating superior risk prediction with the CAC score compared with CIMT alone.

As most modalities assessing subclinical atherosclerosis, CIMT is most useful to assess risk in populations where risk estimation with traditional calculators may underestimate their risk. IMT is uniquely useful in younger cohorts, where lifetime risk may be quite high despite normal CAC score. In addition, although carotid ultrasound evaluating both the carotid IMT and presence of plaque is less predictive than coronary calcium scoring for overall atherosclerotic risk, it is more predictive for stroke risk.[6,31]

The importance of CIMT has continued to decrease with new guideline iterations. The 2018 ACC/AHA guidelines do not assign CIMT a class recommendation but rather mention that it is a weak predictor of overall ASCVD events compared with CAC score.[32] The 2013 ACC/AHA guidelines state that CIMT should not be routinely performed (class III), regardless of initial risk stratification by traditional methods with carotid plaque screening discussed.[33] In contrast, the 2012 ESC and 2010 ACC/AHA guidelines recommend CIMT use (class IIa) for further evaluation of moderate- or intermediate-risk patients.[17] The main limitation of CIMT lies in its operator-dependent nature, requiring skill at image acquisition. It is a relatively fast study, however, adding a few minutes of scan time onto patients who are already undergoing carotid ultrasound. It is also relatively inexpensive and does not require radiation, which is beneficial for younger cohorts.

ANKLE-BRACHIAL index/Toe-BRACHIAL INDEX

ABI is a ratio of the systolic blood pressure measured at the ankle to that measured at the brachial artery. ABIs ranging from 1.0 to 1.4 are considered normal, whereas ABI less than 0.9 and greater than 1.4 are considered abnormal, suggesting vascular disease. Over the past few decades, ABI has proved to be a reliable predictor of cardiovascular disease and death.[30,34–37]

Current 2019 ACC/AHA Guidelines on Primary Prevention of Cardiovascular Disease identify ABI less than 0.9 as a risk enhancing factor to help guide preventative management in borderline and intermediate-risk adults[38,39]; this was illustrated in a study by Ramos and colleagues who investigated patients with asymptomatic peripheral arterial disease (ABI ≤0.95) but without clinically recognized cardiovascular disease (10-year CVD risk average 6.9%).[40] Ramos and colleagues assessed whether statin therapy was associated with a reduction in MACE and mortality over a median 3.6-year follow-up. In statin versus nonstatin users, incidence of MACE was 19.7 and 24.7 events per 1000 person-years, respectively, whereas total mortality rates were 24.8 versus 30.3 per 1000 person-years, respectively.

TBI may be used in lieu of ABI for certain populations such as those with CKD whose ABI may be falsely high due to artery calcification. Guidelines recommend using TBI when ABI is greater than 1.4, as toe arteries are less likely to be calcified. Studies have reported that TBI provides additional or ever better prognostic information than ABI in patients with diabetes and CKD.[41,42] Both ABI and TBI are noninvasive, inexpensive, and radiation-free but are somewhat limited by their operator-dependent nature. Values may also be difficult to interpret values for patients with calcified limbs, on hemodialysis, and with aortic valve disorders.[43]

EMERGING THERAPIES
Fractional Flow Reserve Coronary Computed Tomography

Fractional flow reserve CT processes CCTA to noninvasively estimate fractional flow reserve (FFR). FFR is a commonly used metric in cardiac catheterization, representing

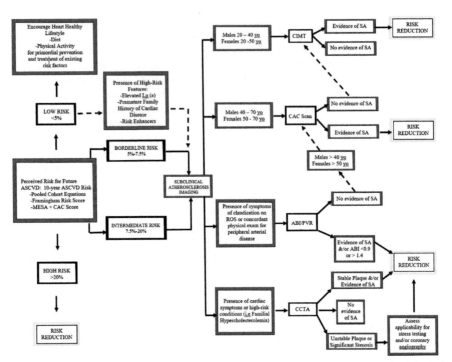

Fig. 2. Proposed flowsheet for risk stratification and subsequent management of subclinical atherosclerosis incorporating imaging modalities discussed in this article. (Reproduced with permission of Soni et al).

a ratio between the pressure in a diseased artery relative to the pressure in a normal artery; this is more traditionally done invasively in the catheterization laboratory using a pressure wire placed across a narrowed artery. HeartFlow FFRCT uses a privatized algorithm replicate that would be found during an FFR assessed invasively.[44] FFRCT should be considered as an option for patients with stable, recent onset chest pain who are offered CCTA as part of an assessment for chest pain, as it may avoid the need for invasive coronary angiography and inappropriate revascularization. The role for FFRCT in risk stratification and primary prevention strategies is an object of ongoing research.

Cardiac Calcification

Cardiac calcifications are frequently encountered on routine echocardiographic examination or CT. Incidental findings of calcific mitral apparatus, aortic valve, and ascending aorta are associated with the clinical manifestation of atherosclerotic disease and are predictive of future cardiovascular events. The ultrasound approach is semiquantitative, summing the numbers of calcified sites and estimating size of each calcification. Studies have found a good relationship between a semiquantitative echocardiographic global calcium scores and quantitative cardiac calcification scores measured on axial CT.[45]

SUMMARY

Imaging assessment of subclinical atherosclerosis has 2 aims: improved risk stratification and more precise approaches to treatment. Imaging allows identification of individuals at higher risk of cardiovascular disease by directly visualizing sequela of the atherosclerotic process. In turn, providers may intensify prevention strategies for those most likely to derive benefit and decrease pharmacotherapies in patients less likely to derive benefit (**Fig. 2**). CAC scans are the most widely used and studied to identify subclinical atherosclerosis, although they have limited utility in younger populations. They are most useful in men older than 40 years and women older than 50 years in whom the results of the CAC would potentially change treatment strategies. CCTA has high prognostic value and might be the best modality for assessing subclinical atherosclerosis, but the incremental increase in predictive value might not be worth the associated radiation and risk of iodinated contrast. In younger cohorts, risk stratification may be enhanced with CIMT, which can be abnormal at a younger age than CAC. ABIs are specific markers for cardiovascular risk, but they have perhaps less value as a sensitive tool for generalized risk assessment. As prognostic data evolve, a more advanced risk calculator will likely incorporate traditional risk factors, novel risk factors, genetic risk, and subclinical atherosclerosis to more accurately assess an individual's risk and guide their treatment accordingly. Ultimately, the goal is to give the right treatments to the right patients.

CLINICS CARE POINTS

- Subclinical atherosclerosis imaging identifies individuals at higher risk of cardiovascular disease, significantly refining the accuracy of risk assessments. With more accurate estimation of risk, subclinical atherosclerosis imaging allows for delivery of preventive treatments to the patients most likely to derive the most benefit.

- CAC scans are the most widely used and studied modality to identify subclinical atherosclerosis. CAC is most useful in men older than 40 years and women older than 50 years with borderline risk profiles, because CAC scores in these populations have the highest likelihood to change the preventative treatment recommendations.

- CCTA has high prognostic value and is the most powerful modality for assessing subclinical atherosclerosis in asymptomatic patients but has only incremental increase in predictive value over CAC alone. CCTA delivers more radiation, has higher associated cost, and carries risk associated with iodinated contrast exposure.

- Risk stratification may be enhanced with CIMT, specifically for men younger than 40 years or women younger than 50 years.

- ABIs are specific markers for cardiovascular risk but are a less sensitive tool for risk assessment.

DISCLOSURE

Dr J.K. Logan and Dr M.P. Ayers have nothing to disclose.

REFERENCES

1. Zipes DP. Braunwald's Heart Disease: A Textbook of Cardiovascular Medicine. 11th edition. 2018.
2. Fernandez-Alvira JM, Fuster V, Pocock S, et al. Predicting subclinical atherosclerosis in low-risk individuals: ideal cardiovascular health score and fuster-BEWAT Score. J Am Coll Cardiol 2017;70(20):2463–73.

3. Ahmadi A, Argulian E, Leipsic J, et al. From subclinical atherosclerosis to plaque progression and acute coronary events: JACC State-of-the-Art review. J Am Coll Cardiol 2019;74(12):1608–17.

4. Hattori K, Ozaki Y, Ismail TF, et al. Impact of statin therapy on plaque characteristics as assessed by serial OCT, grayscale and integrated backscatter-IVUS. JACC Cardiovasc Imaging 2012;5(2):169–77.

5. Inoue K, Motoyama S, Sarai M, et al. Serial coronary CT angiography-verified changes in plaque characteristics as an end point: evaluation of effect of statin intervention. JACC Cardiovasc Imaging 2010;3(7):691–8.

6. Gill EA, Blaha MJ, Guyton JR. JCL roundtable: Coronary artery calcium scoring and other vascular imaging for risk assessment. J Clin Lipidol 2019;13(1):4–14.

7. Agatston AS, Janowitz WR, Hildner FJ, et al. Quantification of coronary artery calcium using ultrafast computed tomography. J Am Coll Cardiol 1990;15(4): 827–32.

8. Hecht HS, Budoff MJ, Berman DS, et al. Coronary artery calcium scanning: clinical paradigms for cardiac risk assessment and treatment. Am Heart J 2006; 151(6):1139–46.

9. Blaha MJ, Cainzos-Achirica M, Greenland P, et al. Role of Coronary Artery Calcium Score of Zero and Other Negative Risk Markers for Cardiovascular Disease: The Multi-Ethnic Study of Atherosclerosis (MESA). Circulation 2016;133(9): 849–58.

10. Arnett DK, Blumenthal RS, Albert MA, et al. 2019 ACC/AHA Guideline on the Primary Prevention of Cardiovascular Disease: Executive Summary: A Report of the American College of Cardiology/American Heart Association Task Force on Clinical Practice Guidelines. J Am Coll Cardiol 2019;74(10):1376–414.

11. Polonsky TS, McClelland RL, Jorgensen NW, et al. Coronary artery calcium score and risk classification for coronary heart disease prediction. JAMA 2010;303(16): 1610–6.

12. Detrano R, Guerci AD, Carr JJ, et al. Coronary calcium as a predictor of coronary events in four racial or ethnic groups. N Engl J Med 2008;358(13):1336–45.

13. McClelland RL, Chung H, Detrano R, et al. Distribution of coronary artery calcium by race, gender, and age: results from the Multi-Ethnic Study of Atherosclerosis (MESA). Circulation 2006;113(1):30–7.

14. Shaw LJ, Min JK, Nasir K, et al. Sex differences in calcified plaque and long-term cardiovascular mortality: observations from the CAC Consortium. Eur Heart J 2018;39(41):3727–35.

15. Naghavi M, Falk E, Hecht HS, et al. From vulnerable plaque to vulnerable patient– Part III: Executive summary of the Screening for Heart Attack Prevention and Education (SHAPE) Task Force report. Am J Cardiol 2006;98(2A):2H–15H.

16. Greenland P, Alpert JS, Beller GA, et al. 2010 ACCF/AHA guideline for assessment of cardiovascular risk in asymptomatic adults: a report of the American College of Cardiology Foundation/American Heart Association Task Force on Practice Guidelines. J Am Coll Cardiol 2010;56(25):e50–103.

17. Perk J, De Backer G, Gohlke H, et al. European Guidelines on cardiovascular disease prevention in clinical practice (version 2012). The Fifth Joint Task Force of the European Society of Cardiology and Other Societies on Cardiovascular Disease Prevention in Clinical Practice (constituted by representatives of nine societies and by invited experts). Eur Heart J 2012;33(13):1635–701.

18. Abu Daya H, Hage FG. Guidelines in review: ACC/AATS/AHA/ASE/ASNC/SCAI/ SCCT/STS 2017 appropriate use criteria for coronary revascularization in patients with stable ischemic heart disease. J Nucl Cardiol 2017;24(5):1793–9.

19. Abdelrahman KM, Chen MY, Dey AK, et al. Coronary computed tomography angiography from clinical uses to emerging technologies: JACC State-of-the-Art review. J Am Coll Cardiol 2020;76(10):1226–43.

20. Abbara S, Blanke P, Maroules CD, et al. SCCT guidelines for the performance and acquisition of coronary computed tomographic angiography: a report of the society of Cardiovascular Computed Tomography Guidelines Committee: Endorsed by the North American Society for Cardiovascular Imaging (NASCI). J Cardiovasc Comput Tomogr 2016;10(6):435–49.

21. Knuuti J, Wijns W, Saraste A, et al. 2019 ESC Guidelines for the diagnosis and management of chronic coronary syndromes. Eur Heart J 2020;41(3):407–77.

22. SCOT-HEART Investigators. CT coronary angiography in patients with suspected angina due to coronary heart disease (SCOT-HEART): an open-label, parallel-group, multicentre trial. Lancet 2015;385(9985):2383–91.

23. Investigators S-H, Newby DE, Adamson PD, et al. Coronary CT Angiography and 5-Year Risk of Myocardial Infarction. N Engl J Med 2018;379(10):924–33.

24. Hoffmann U, Ferencik M, Udelson JE, et al. Prognostic Value of Noninvasive Cardiovascular Testing in Patients With Stable Chest Pain: Insights From the PROMISE Trial (Prospective Multicenter Imaging Study for Evaluation of Chest Pain). Circulation 2017;135(24):2320–32.

25. Douglas PS, Hoffmann U, Patel MR, et al. Outcomes of anatomical versus functional testing for coronary artery disease. N Engl J Med 2015;372(14):1291–300.

26. Cho I, Chang HJ, Sung JM, et al. Coronary computed tomographic angiography and risk of all-cause mortality and nonfatal myocardial infarction in subjects without chest pain syndrome from the CONFIRM Registry (coronary CT angiography evaluation for clinical outcomes: an international multicenter registry). Circulation 2012;126(3):304–13.

27. Lee SE, Chang HJ, Sung JM, et al. Effects of Statins on Coronary Atherosclerotic Plaques: The PARADIGM Study. JACC Cardiovasc Imaging 2018;11(10):1475–84.

28. Willeit P, Tschiderer L, Allara E, et al. Carotid Intima-Media Thickness Progression as Surrogate Marker for Cardiovascular Risk: Meta-Analysis of 119 Clinical Trials Involving 100 667 Patients. Circulation 2020;142(7):621–42.

29. Nambi V, Chambless L, Folsom AR, et al. Carotid intima-media thickness and presence or absence of plaque improves prediction of coronary heart disease risk: the ARIC (Atherosclerosis Risk In Communities) study. J Am Coll Cardiol 2010;55(15):1600–7.

30. Polak JF, Szklo M, O'Leary DH. Carotid Intima-Media Thickness Score, Positive Coronary Artery Calcium Score, and Incident Coronary Heart Disease: The Multi-Ethnic Study of Atherosclerosis. J Am Heart Assoc 2017;6(1). https://doi.org/10.1161/JAHA.116.004612.

31. Gepner AD, Young R, Delaney JA, et al. Comparison of Carotid Plaque Score and Coronary Artery Calcium Score for Predicting Cardiovascular Disease Events: The Multi-Ethnic Study of Atherosclerosis. J Am Heart Assoc 2017;6(2). https://doi.org/10.1161/JAHA.116.005179.

32. Lloyd-Jones DM, Braun LT, Ndumele CE, et al. Use of Risk Assessment Tools to Guide Decision-Making in the Primary Prevention of Atherosclerotic Cardiovascular Disease: A Special Report From the American Heart Association and American College of Cardiology. J Am Coll Cardiol 2019;73(24):3153–67.

33. Goff DC Jr, Lloyd-Jones DM, Bennett G, et al. 2013 ACC/AHA guideline on the assessment of cardiovascular risk: a report of the American College of

Cardiology/American Heart Association Task Force on Practice Guidelines. J Am Coll Cardiol 2014;63(25 Pt B):2935–59.

34. Aboyans V, Criqui MH, Abraham P, et al. Measurement and interpretation of the ankle-brachial index: a scientific statement from the American Heart Association. Circulation 2012;126(24):2890–909.

35. Doobay AV, Anand SS. Sensitivity and specificity of the ankle-brachial index to predict future cardiovascular outcomes: a systematic review. Arterioscler Thromb Vasc Biol 2005;25(7):1463–9.

36. Geisel MH, Bauer M, Hennig F, et al. Comparison of coronary artery calcification, carotid intima-media thickness and ankle-brachial index for predicting 10-year incident cardiovascular events in the general population. Eur Heart J 2017; 38(23):1815–22.

37. Ohkuma T, Ninomiya T, Tomiyama H, et al. Ankle-brachial index measured by oscillometry is predictive for cardiovascular disease and premature death in the Japanese population: an individual participant data meta-analysis. Atherosclerosis 2018;275:141–8.

38. Papageorgiou N, Briasoulis A, Androulakis E, et al. Imaging subclinical atherosclerosis: where do we stand? Curr Cardiol Rev 2017;13(1):47–55.

39. Fowkes FG, Price JF, Stewart MC, et al. Aspirin for prevention of cardiovascular events in a general population screened for a low ankle brachial index: a randomized controlled trial. JAMA 2010;303(9):841–8.

40. Ramos R, Garcia-Gil M, Comas-Cufi M, et al. Statins for prevention of cardiovascular events in a low-risk population with low ankle brachial index. J Am Coll Cardiol 2016;67(6):630–40.

41. Hyun S, Forbang NI, Allison MA, et al. Ankle-brachial index, toe-brachial index, and cardiovascular mortality in persons with and without diabetes mellitus. J Vasc Surg 2014;60(2):390–5.

42. Kamath TP, Prasad R, Allison MA, et al. Association of Ankle-Brachial and Toe-Brachial Indexes With Mortality in Patients With CKD. Kidney Med 2020;2(1): 68–75.

43. Ato D. Pitfalls in the ankle-brachial index and brachial-ankle pulse wave velocity. Vasc Health Risk Manag 2018;14:41–62.

44. Mahmoudi M, Nicholas Z, Nuttall J, et al. Fractional flow reserve derived from computed tomography coronary angiography in the assessment and management of stable chest pain: rationale and design of the FORECAST Trial. Cardiovasc Revasc Med 2020;21(7):890–6.

45. Faggiano P, Dasseni N, Gaibazzi N, et al. Cardiac calcification as a marker of subclinical atherosclerosis and predictor of cardiovascular events: a review of the evidence. Eur J Prev Cardiol 2019;26(11):1191–204.

Drug Interactions

What Are Important Drug Interactions for the Most Commonly Used Medications in Preventive Cardiology?

Aziz Hammoud, MD[a], Michael D. Shapiro, DO, MCR[a,b,c,*]

KEYWORDS

• Drug interactions • Preventive cardiology • Statins

KEY POINTS

• Drug interactions are a major concern in preventive cardiology because of the widespread use of statins.
• Clinically significant statin interactions are predictable and preventable with an understanding of statin pharmacokinetics and how they differ from statin to statin.
• Novel lipid-lowering therapies, such as proprotein convertase subtilisin/kexin type 9 inhibition with monoclonal antibodies or small interfering RNAs, have favorable drug interaction profiles.

INTRODUCTION

Drug interactions are defined as 2 or more substances that interact in such a way that the effectiveness or toxicity of 1 or more substance is modified. Many interactions are theoretic or clinically trivial; however, some may have serious or life-threatening consequences.[1] They are estimated to cause approximately 2.8% of all hospitalizations annually in the United States, representing more than 245,000 hospitalizations and costing the health care system $1.3 billion.[2] Moreover, the actual incidence of hospitalization secondary to clinically significant drug interactions is likely to be underestimated because medication-related issues are reported more commonly as adverse drug reactions and often confounded by complex underlying disease states.[3] The

[a] Section on Cardiovascular Medicine, Department of Medicine, Wake Forest University School of Medicine, Winston-Salem, NC, USA; [b] Section on Cardiovascular Medicine, Department of Internal Medicine, Wake Forest University School of Medicine, Winston-Salem, NC, USA; [c] Center for Prevention of Cardiovascular Disease, Medical Center Boulevard, Winston Salem, NC 27157, USA
* Corresponding author. Section on Cardiovascular Medicine, Department of Internal Medicine, Wake Forest University School of Medicine, Winston-Salem, NC.
E-mail address: mdshapir@wakehealth.edu

Med Clin N Am 106 (2022) 389–399
https://doi.org/10.1016/j.mcna.2021.11.013
0025-7125/22/© 2021 Elsevier Inc. All rights reserved.

aging population, high prevalence of chronic diseases, and polypharmacy are some factors closely associated with potential drug interactions.[4]

Several types of drug interactions exist: drug-drug, drug-food, drug-supplement, and drug-patient.[5] Drug-drug interactions—the focus of this review—can be pharmacokinetic or pharmacodynamic in nature. Pharmacokinetics involve the effects of one drug on the absorption, distribution, metabolism, or excretion of another drug, which can result in changes in serum drug concentrations and clinical response.[6] Pharmacokinetic drug interactions frequently involve isoenzymes of the hepatic cytochrome P450 (CYP) system and membrane transporters, such as organic anion transporting polypeptides (OATPs) and P-glycoprotein (P-gp), also known as multidrug resistance-associated protein (MRP) 1. Pharmacodynamics are related to the pharmacologic activity of the interacting drugs, and the outcome is an amplification or decrease in the therapeutic effects or side-effects of a specific drug in an additive, a synergistic, or an antagonistic fashion.[3]

Clinically significant drug interactions usually are preventable. To optimize patient safety, providers should understand the mechanisms, magnitude, and potential consequences of any given drug interaction. This article provides an overview of important drug interactions for commonly used medications in preventive cardiology, with an emphasis on clinically important drug-drug interactions involving conventional lipid-lowering agents.

DISCUSSION
Statin Pharmacology

One in 4 Americans greater than 40 years of age takes a statin to reduce the risk of atherosclerotic cardiovascular disease (ASCVD).[7] Statins reduce hepatic cholesterol synthesis by competitively blocking 3-hydroxy-3-methylglutaryl coenzyme A reductase, thereby leading to increased cell surface low-density lipoprotein (LDL) receptor expression and clearance of LDL-cholesterol (LDL-C) from the bloodstream.[8] The most effective statins produce a mean reduction in LDL-C of 55% to 60% at the maximum dosage.[7] They also may exhibit non–lipid-related pleiotropic effects, including improved endothelial function, atherosclerotic plaque stabilization, anti-inflammatory, immunomodulatory, and antithrombotic effects.[9] They reduce morbidity and mortality in individuals with ASCVD and thus are a mainstay of therapy for these individuals. The 2018 American Heart Association/American College of Cardiology Guideline on the Management of Blood Cholesterol also recommends statins for individuals with diabetes mellitus, individuals with LDL-C greater than or equal to 190 mg/dL, and adults in primary prevention with an estimated 10-year ASCVD risk greater than or equal to 7.5%.[10]

Statin toxicity or intolerance presents most commonly as statin-associated muscle symptoms (SAMs)—muscle aches or pains reported during statin therapy but not necessarily caused by the statin. The incidence of SAMs is 10% to 15% of patients in observational studies, as high as 30% according to clinic data, and 1.5% to 5% in randomized controlled trials, which likely is an underestimation because most studies exclude patients with a history of statin intolerance.[8] Myopathy, defined as unexplained muscle pain or weakness accompanied by increases in creatine kinase above 10 times the upper limit of normal, is the hallmark adverse effect of statins; however, it is rare, occurring in less than 1 in 1000 patients treated with maximum recommended doses and with an even lower risk at lower doses. Approximately 1 in 10,000 patients experience rhabdomyolysis, a severe form of myopathy leading to acute renal failure because of myoglobinuria. Prompt cessation of therapy usually reverses statin myopathy, whose mechanism remains unknown. Hepatotoxicity is also associated with statins in approximately 1% of patients, usually in the form of an asymptomatic and temporary transaminitis without histopathologic changes and inconsistent with true liver injury. Monitoring transaminases is not useful in preventing clinically significant statin hepatotoxicity, which occurs in approximately 0.001% of patients.[7]

The metabolic pathway of statins is summarized in **Fig. 1**. Statin pharmacokinetics are highly dependent on membrane transporters that can be broadly classified into uptake and efflux transporters. Uptake transporters belong to the solute-linked carrier (SLC) superfamily and are responsible for the movement of substrates into cells.[6] In contrast, efflux transporters belong to the adenosine triphosphate–binding cassette (ABC) superfamily and are responsible for the movement of substrates out of cells. Statins enter portal circulation through enterocytes by both passive and active transport via OATP1B3 and OATP1A2.[11] P-gp, breast cancer resistance protein (BCRP), and MRP2 also are expressed on the apical membrane of enterocytes and modulate statin absorption. Enterocyte CYP isoenzymes may metabolize some statins before they are absorbed. OATP1B1 and OATP1B3 are expressed on the basolateral membrane of hepatocytes and are involved in hepatic uptake of statins. In the liver, statins undergo phase I oxidation (mediated by CYP isoenzymes) and phase II glucuronidation (mediated by uridine 5′-diphospho-glucuronosyltransferases [UGT]). The main pathway of elimination is biliary excretion mediated by P-gp, BCRP, and MRP2 expressed on the bile canicular membrane.

The pharmacokinetic properties of statins are complex, variable from statin to statin, and central in understanding statin interactions (**Table 1**). Except for simvastatin and lovastatin, which are given as prodrugs, all statins are administered in the active hydroxyl acid form.[6] Systemic bioavailability for all statins is considered low, ranging from less than 5% for simvastatin and lovastatin to 51% for pitavastatin. All statins except pravastatin and rosuvastatin are considered lipophilic, and most statins consequently are highly protein bound. Lipophilic statins require a greater degree of

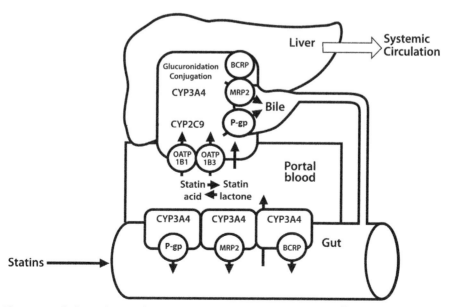

Fig. 1. Metabolic pathway of statins. (*Adapted from* Neuvonen et al.[13])

Table 1
Pharmacokinetic variables of marketed statins in the United States

Variable	Atorvastatin	Fluvastatin	Lovastatin	Pitavastatin	Pravastatin	Rosuvastatin	Simvastatin
Prodrug	No	No	Yes	No	No	No	Yes
High lipid solubility	Yes	Yes	Yes	Yes	No	No	Yes
T_{max} (h)	1.0–2.0	<1.0	2.0–4.0	1.0	1.0–1.5	3.0–5.0	4.0
$T_{1/2}$ (h)	14	<3	2	12	2	19	2
Bioavailability (%)	14	24	<5	51	17	20	<5
Protein binding (%)	>98	98	>95	99	50	88	95
Major CYP metabolism	CYP3A4	CYP2C9 CYP2C8	CYP3A4	CYP2C9 CYP2C8 (minor)	None	CYP2C9 (minor)	CYP3A4
Major transporters	P-gp OATP1B1 OATP2B1 BCRP	OATP1B1 OATP1B3 OATP2B1 BCRP	P-gp OATP1B1 BCRP	P-gp OATP1B1 OATP1B3 OATP2B1 BCRP	OATP1B1 OATP1B3 OATP2B1 BCRP	OATP1B1 OATP1B3 OAT2B1 BCRP NTCP	P-gp OATP1B1
Systemic active metabolites	Yes[2]	No	Yes[4]	No	No	Minimal	Yes[3]
Renal excretion (%)	<2	<6	10	15	20	10	13

Abbreviations: T_{max}, amount of time that a drug is present at the maximum concentration in serum; NTCP, sodium-taurocholate cotransporting polypeptide; $T_{1/2}$, drug half-life.[6]

metabolism to convert the statin into water-soluble salts and conjugates that are eliminated from the body. Simvastatin and lovastatin undergo significant CYP3A4 metabolism, and atorvastatin undergoes a lesser amount as one of its minor metabolic pathways. In contrast, fluvastatin, pitavastatin, and rosuvastatin undergo significant CYP2C9 metabolism. Pravastatin is the only statin that does not undergo CYP metabolism. The overall dependence of statin metabolites on renal elimination is modest, with pravastatin the highest at 20% and atorvastatin the lowest at less than 2%.[12]

Clinically Significant Statin-Drug Interactions

Drugs that inhibit the CYP3A4 enzyme can interfere with the metabolism of simvastatin, lovastatin, and, to a lesser extent, atorvastatin. The principal drugs that inhibit CYP3A4 are the azole antifungals ketoconazole and itraconazole (but not fluconazole); the macrolide antibiotics clarithromycin and erythromycin (but not azithromycin); the human immunodeficiency virus protease inhibitors; the antiarrhythmics amiodarone and dronedarone; and the non-dihydropyridine calcium channel blockers diltiazem and verapamil (no effect on atorvastatin).[13,14] Current Food and Drug Administration (FDA) labeling advises that the dose of simvastatin not exceed 10 mg daily and the dose of lovastatin not exceed 20 mg daily when coprescribed with diltiazem or verapamil in adults (**Table 2**).[3] Similarly, the FDA-approved product labeling for amlodipine, a substrate of CYP3A4, indicates that there may be an increased risk of muscle-related toxicity when combined with simvastatin and recommends a dose limit of 20 mg daily when coprescribed. Furthermore, FDA labeling recommends a dose limit of simvastatin, 20 mg daily, and of lovastatin, 40 mg daily, when coprescribed with amiodarone and a dose limit of simvastatin, 10 mg daily, and lovastatin, 20 mg daily, when coprescribed with dronedarone.[3]

Some drugs that inhibit CYP2C9 are azole antifungals, omeprazole, cimetidine, and tolbutamide. Although these drugs theoretically may interact with fluvastatin, few clinically important fluvastatin interactions have been reported. The most significant fluvastatin interaction occurs with fluconazole, and prescribing information for fluvastatin advises a dose limit of 20 mg daily when used with fluconazole. This caution does not extend to pitavastatin, which also relies on CYP2C9 metabolism. CYP2C9 plays an important role in the metabolism of warfarin, a vitamin K antagonist and commonly used oral anticoagulant, yet it has no clinically significant interactions with statins.[3] Until more definitive data are available, the international normalized ratio (INR) should be monitored more closely after the initiation of a statin or any change in statin dose.

Some foods and supplements also have been associated with clinically significant statin interactions. For instance, grapefruit products contain bergamottin, a natural furanocoumarin, which can inhibit intestinal CYP3A4 and increase systemic statin exposure in a dose-dependent manner that increases with the concentration and volume of grapefruit consumed.[6] According to FDA labeling, grapefruit juice should be avoided with lovastatin, and excessive consumption of grapefruit juice (>1 L/d) should be avoided with simvastatin and atorvastatin. Alternatively, any of the statins that are not metabolized by CYP3A4 may be safely used with grapefruit products. St. John's wort, a common supplement for depression, induces CYP3A4 and P-gp.[15] It decreases the metabolism of simvastatin and possibly atorvastatin but not the others in the class.[6] Health care providers also should be aware of red yeast rice extract, a popular cholesterol-lowering supplement. Red rice yeast contains varying amounts of monacolin K, which structurally is identical to lovastatin. Thus, patients on statins should be advised to avoid red yeast rice products.

Table 2
Clinically significant statin-drug interactions and recommended dose limits

Drug	Atorvastatin	Fluvastatin	Lovastatin	Pitavastatin	Pravastatin	Rosuvastatin	Simvastatin
Amiodarone			40 mg/d				20 mg/d
Amlodipine			20 mg/d				20 mg/d
Colchicine	Caution	Caution	Caution	Caution	Caution	Caution	Caution
Conivaptan	Avoid	Avoid	Avoid	Avoid	Avoid	Avoid	Avoid
Calcineurin inhibitors	10 mg/d	40 mg/d	Avoid	Avoid	20 mg/d	5 mg/d	Avoid
mTOR inhibitors	10 mg/d	40 mg/d	Avoid	Avoid	20 mg/d	5 mg/d	Avoid
Diltiazem			20 mg/d				10 mg/d
Dronedarone			10 mg/d				10 mg/d
Gemfibrozil	Avoid	Avoid	Avoid	Avoid	Avoid	Avoid	Avoid
Ranolazine			20 mg/d				20 mg/d
Ticagrelor			40 mg/d				40 mg/d
Verapamil			20 mg/d				10 mg/d
Warfarin	Monitor INR more closely after initiation of a statin or change in statin dose.						
Ketoconazole			Avoid				Avoid
Fluconazole		20 mg/d					
Posaconazole			Avoid				Avoid
Itraconazole	20 mg/d						
Clarithromycin	20 mg/d						
Erythromycin				1 mg/d			
Danazol			Avoid				Avoid
Digoxin	Coadministration is reasonable, if clinically indicated.						
Niacin	Limit dose of niacin to 1 g/d						
Bempedoic acid					40 mg/d		20 mg/d

Atazanavir + ritonavir		Avoid	10 mg/d	Avoid
Darunavir + ritonavir	20 mg/d	Avoid		Avoid
Fosamprenavir + ritonavir	20 mg/d	Avoid		Avoid
Lopinavir + ritonavir	Caution	Avoid		Avoid
Nelfinavir	40 mg/d	Avoid	10 mg/d	Avoid
Tipranavir + ritonavir	Avoid	Avoid		Avoid
Saquinavir + ritonavir	20 mg/d	Avoid		Avoid

Dose limits derived from FDA labels. Empty cells represent the absence of conclusive data on clinically significant interactions. Cells with numbers represent the dose limit based on drug labeling. "Avoid" indicates that the combination is contraindicated. Caution indicates that the combination may be considered with close monitoring.

Statins commonly are coprescribed with immunosuppressants, especially among heart transplant recipients. Current guidelines strongly recommend initiation of statins within 1 week to 2 weeks of heart transplantation, irrespective of lipid profiles, because statins have been associated with a reduction in mortality, hemodynamically significant rejection episodes, and incidence of coronary vasculopathy.[16,17] Calcineurin inhibitors, such as cyclosporine and tacrolimus, are metabolized extensively by hepatic and intestinal CYP3A4, both inhibitors and substrates of P-gp, and inhibitors of OATP1B1 and OATP1B3.[13] As a result, calcineurin inhibitors are predisposed to potential pharmacokinetic interactions with all statins. Additionally, numerous cases of rhabdomyolysis have occurred with concomitant use of cyclosporine and various statins, except for fluvastatin.[13] Similarly, sirolimus and everolimus have extensive hepatic and intestinal metabolism by CYP3A4 and P-gp. Few data exist, however, on the interactions between mammalian target of rapamycin inhibitors and statins (mTOR). Combination therapy of any of these immunosuppressants with lovastatin, simvastatin, or pitavastatin potentially is harmful and should be avoided. Daily doses of fluvastatin, pravastatin, rosuvastatin, and atorvastatin should be limited to 40 mg, 20 mg, 5 mg, and 10 mg daily, respectively, when combined with calcineurin inhibitors or mTOR inhibitors.[3]

Drug Interactions with Other Lipid-lowering Therapies

Coadministration of statins with a fibrate may be warranted for treatment of severe hypertriglyceridemia or complex dyslipidemias.[3] In the United States, gemfibrozil, fenofibrate, and fenofibric acid are the only fibrates approved for clinical use. Both statins and fibrates have been independently associated with a risk of muscle-related toxicity, and the statin-fibrate combination therapy increases this risk.[18,19] Gemfibrozil, but not fenofibrate, adversely affects the pharmacokinetics of most statins due to several mechanisms, including inhibition of OATP1B1-mediated hepatic uptake, CYP2C8 metabolism, and glucuronidation and subsequent lactonization by UGT1A1 and UGT1A3 enzymes.[20,21] Gemfibrozil and its glucuronide metabolite also are substrates of CYP3A4. The net result of these interactions is a higher concentration of active, open acid statins in the systemic circulation and a greater risk of adverse effects. Thus, the combination of any statin and gemfibrozil should be avoided. When statin-fibrate combination therapy is indicated, fenofibrate is preferred.[3]

Other LDL-C–lowering agents that may be coadministered with statins are ezetimibe and bempedoic acid. Initially approved in the United States in 2002, ezetimibe inhibits absorption of cholesterol in the small intestine by targeting the sterol transporter, Niemann-Pick C1-Like 1.[22] It is metabolized primarily in the small intestine and liver via glucuronide conjugation (phase II reaction) with subsequent biliary and renal excretion.[23] Ezetimibe and statins can be used together without significant concern for adverse interactions; however, the current FDA labeling warns of increased risk of myopathy and cholelithiasis when combining ezetimibe and fibrates. In February 2020, the FDA approved bempedoic acid for treatment of adults with heterozygous familial hypercholesteremia or established ASCVD who require additional lowering of LDL-C.[24] Bempedoic acid lowers LDL-C by inhibiting adenosine triphosphate citrate lyase, a key enzyme in the cholesterol biosynthesis pathway that acts upstream of 3-hydroxy-3-methylglutaryl coenzyme A reductase.[25] It is a prodrug that requires activation by the enzyme very-long-chain acyl–coenzyme A synthetase 1, which is present in the liver but absent in most peripheral tissue, including muscle. Bempedoic acid and its metabolite are converted by UGT2B7 to glucuronide conjugates that are inactive.[24] Concurrent use of bempedoic acid with greater than 20 mg of simvastatin or 40 mg of pravastatin increases the risk of myopathies and should be avoided, according to the FDA label. Additionally, a combination of statins or bempedoic acid with ezetimibe may offer synergistic lipid-lowering activity compared with monotherapy because of their complementary mechanisms of actions that couple inhibition of hepatic cholesterol synthesis and inhibition intestinal cholesterol absorption.[26–28]

There is little concern for drug interactions among novel lipid-lowering therapies targeting proprotein convertase subtilisin/kexin type 9 (PCSK9), an enzyme that binds LDL receptors, leading to their degradation and subsequently higher plasma LDL-C levels, given their novel mechanisms of action. Evolocumab and alirocumab are FDA-approved fully human monoclonal antibodies that inhibit plasma PCSK9. Although statins stimulate PCSK9 through an increased release of sterol regulatory element-binding protein 2, the percent of LDL-C reduction with PCSK9monoclonal antibodies is independent of statin use.[29,30] An alternative approach to antagonizing PCSK9leverages small interfering RNAs that prevent intracellular translation of PCSK9 messenger RNA to protein. Inclisiran, a long-acting, synthetic, small interfering RNA directed against PCSK9 messenger RNA conjugated to triantennary N-acetylgalactosamine carbohydrates, which bind liver-expressed asialoglycoprotein receptors with high affinity, is associated with LDL-C reduction that rivals the therapeutic monoclonal antibodies.[31] Inclisiran was approved by the European Commission in December 2020, for the treatment of adults with primary hypercholesteremia or mixed dyslipidemia and currently is awaiting regulatory approval in the United States.

Principles of Drug Interaction Avoidance

Health care providers should be aware of serious drug interactions and tailor drug combinations to avoid them. General strategies for reducing the risk of drug-drug interactions include minimizing the number of drugs prescribed, re-evaluating therapy on a regular basis, considering nonpharmacologic options when possible, monitoring for signs and symptoms of toxicity and/or effectiveness, and adjusting drug doses or administration times, when indicated.[1] Software within the electronic health record that detects and alerts providers of potential drug interactions lowers the risk of some drug interactions at the cost of alert fatigue.[32] Additionally, medication review and reconciliation by a pharmacist may reduce the risk of clinically significant drug interactions.

SUMMARY

Many of the most common drug interactions within preventive cardiology involve statins. These interactions often are predictable by understanding the pharmacokinetics of this class of medications. The variation in their pharmacokinetics allows providers to tailor drug combinations to avoid clinically significant interactions. Although statins will continue to be the backbone of lipid-lowering therapy for primary and secondary ASCVD prevention, novel lipid-lowering agents may offer more favorable drug interaction profiles.

CLINICS CARE POINTS

- Statins are the primary lipid-lowering therapy but have several drug interactions dictated by their metabolism.
- The pharmacokinetics of statins differ from statin to statin, so drug combinations can be tailored in such a way to avoid clinically significant interactions.

- Simvastatin and lovastatin have the most documented drug interactions because of their CYP3A4 metabolism.
- Providers should screen patients for possible drug-food and drug-supplement interactions with statins.
- Drug interaction screening using the electronic health record and pharmacists may help prevent clinically significant drug interactions.
- Novel lipid-lowering therapies often have favorable drug interaction profiles.

DISCLOSURE

A. Hammoud has nothing to disclose. M.D. Shapiro reports scientific advisory activities with Amgen, Esperion, and Novartis.

REFERENCES

1. Carpenter M, Berry H, Pelletier AL. Clinically Relevant Drug-Drug Interactions in Primary Care. Am Fam Physician 2019;99(9):558–64.
2. Nikolic B, Jankovic S, Stojanov O, et al. Prevalence and predictors of potential drug-drug interactions. Cent Eur J Med 2014;9:348–56.
3. Wiggins BS, Saseen JJ, Page RL 2nd, et al. Recommendations for Management of Clinically Significant Drug-Drug Interactions With Statins and Select Agents Used in Patients With Cardiovascular Disease: A Scientific Statement From the American Heart Association. Circulation 2016;134(21):e468–95.
4. Sánchez-fidalgo S, Guzmán-ramos MI, Galván-banqueri M, et al. Prevalence of drug interactions in elderly patients with multimorbidity in primary care. Int J Clin Pharm 2017;39(2):343–53.
5. Mallet L, Spinewine A, Huang A. The challenge of managing drug interactions in elderly people. Lancet 2007;370(9582):185–91.
6. Kellick KA, Bottorff M, Toth PP. The National Lipid Association's Safety Task F. A clinician's guide to statin drug-drug interactions. J Clin Lipidol 2014;8(3 Suppl):S30–46.
7. Newman CB, Preiss D, Tobert JA, et al. Statin Safety and Associated Adverse Events: A Scientific Statement From the American Heart Association. Arterioscler Thromb Vasc Biol 2019;39(2):e38–81.
8. Ward NC, Watts GF, Eckel RH. Statin Toxicity. Circ Res 2019;124(2):328–50.
9. Kavalipati N, Shah J, Ramakrishan A, et al. Pleiotropic effects of statins. Indian J Endocrinol Metab 2015;19(5):554–62.
10. Arnett DK, Blumenthal RS, Albert MA, et al. 2019 ACC/AHA Guideline on the Primary Prevention of Cardiovascular Disease: Executive Summary: A Report of the American College of Cardiology/American Heart Association Task Force on Clinical Practice Guidelines. Circulation 2019;140(11):e563–95.
11. Whirl-Carrillo M, Huddart R, Gong L, et al. An evidence-based framework for evaluating pharmacogenomics knowledge for personalized medicine. Clin Pharmacol Ther 2021;110(3):563–72.
12. Ballantyne C. Clinical Lipidology: A Companion to Braunwald's Heart Disease. 2014. Available at: https://www.elsevier.com/books/clinical-lipidology-a-companion-to-braunwalds-heart-disease/ballantyne/978-0-323-28786-9.
13. Neuvonen PJ, Niemi M, Backman JT. Drug interactions with lipid-lowering drugs: Mechanisms and clinical relevance. Clin Pharmacol Ther 2006;80(6):565–81.

14. Bellosta S, Corsini A. Statin drug interactions and related adverse reactions. Expert Opin Drug Saf 2012;11(6):933–46.

15. Holtzman CW, Wiggins BS, Spinler SA. Role of P-glycoprotein in statin drug interactions. Pharmacotherapy 2006;26(11):1601–7.

16. Costanzo MR, Dipchand A, Starling R, et al. The International Society of Heart and Lung Transplantation Guidelines for the care of heart transplant recipients. J Heart Lung Transplant 2010;29(8):914–56.

17. Vallakati A, Reddy S, Dunlap ME, et al. Impact of Statin Use After Heart Transplantation. Circ Heart Fail 2016;9(10):e003265.

18. Farnier M. Safety review of combination drugs for hyperlipidemia. Expert Opin Drug Saf 2011;10(3):363–71.

19. Graham DJ, Staffa JA, Shatin D, et al. Incidence of hospitalized rhabdomyolysis in patients treated with lipid-lowering drugs. Jama 2004;292(21):2585–90.

20. Shitara Y, Hirano M, Sato H, et al. Gemfibrozil and its glucuronide inhibit the organic anion transporting polypeptide 2 (OATP2/OATP1B1:SLC21A6)-mediated hepatic uptake and CYP2C8-mediated metabolism of cerivastatin: analysis of the mechanism of the clinically relevant drug-drug interaction between cerivastatin and gemfibrozil. J Pharmacol Exp Ther 2004;311(1):228–36.

21. Prueksaritanont T, Tang C, Qiu Y, et al. Effects of fibrates on metabolism of statins in human hepatocytes. Drug Metab Dispos 2002;30(11):1280–7.

22. Jia L, Betters JL, Yu L. Niemann-pick C1-like 1 (NPC1L1) protein in intestinal and hepatic cholesterol transport. Annu Rev Physiol 2011;73:239–59.

23. Kosoglou T, Statkevich P, Johnson-Levonas AO, et al. Ezetimibe: a review of its metabolism, pharmacokinetics and drug interactions. Clin Pharmacokinet 2005; 44(5):467–94.

24. Nguyen D, Du N, Sulaica EM, et al. Bempedoic Acid: A New Drug for an Old Problem. Ann Pharmacother 2021;55(2):246–51.

25. Ray KK, Bays HE, Catapano AL, et al. Safety and Efficacy of Bempedoic Acid to Reduce LDL Cholesterol. N Engl J Med 2019;380(11):1022–32.

26. Gagné C, Gaudet D, Bruckert E. Efficacy and safety of ezetimibe coadministered with atorvastatin or simvastatin in patients with homozygous familial hypercholesterolemia. Circulation 2002;105(21):2469–75.

27. Kerzner B, Corbelli J, Sharp S, et al. Efficacy and safety of ezetimibe coadministered with lovastatin in primary hypercholesterolemia. Am J Cardiol 2003;91(4): 418–24.

28. Khan SU, Michos ED. Bempedoic acid and ezetimibe - better together. Eur J Prev Cardiol 2020;27(6):590–2.

29. Mayne J, Dewpura T, Raymond A, et al. Plasma PCSK9 levels are significantly modified by statins and fibrates in humans. Lipids Health Dis 2008;7(1):22.

30. Robinson JG, Nedergaard BS, Rogers WJ, et al. Effect of evolocumab or ezetimibe added to moderate- or high-intensity statin therapy on LDL-C lowering in patients with hypercholesterolemia: the LAPLACE-2 randomized clinical trial. Jama 2014;311(18):1870–82.

31. German CA, Shapiro MD. Small Interfering RNA Therapeutic Inclisiran: A New Approach to Targeting PCSK9. BioDrugs 2020;34(1):1–9.

32. Yeh ML, Chang YJ, Wang PY, et al. Physicians' responses to computerized drug-drug interaction alerts for outpatients. Comput Methods Programs Biomed 2013; 111(1):17–25.

Race and Modifiable Factors Influencing Cardiovascular Disease

Alvis Coleman Headen, BS[a,1],
Andrew Siaw-Asamoah, BA, MPhil[a,1],
Howard M. Julien, MD, MPH, ML[a,b,c,1,*]

KEYWORDS

- Hypertension • Hyperlipidemia • Race • Health care disparities

KEY POINTS

- Cardiovascular disease remains the leading cause of death in the United States with differences in cardiovascular disease mortality between Black and white Americans first manifesting in young and middle-aged adults.
- A modern approach to mitigating the impact of cardiovascular disease on Americans demands not only an understanding of modifiable conditions that contribute to its development but also a greater appreciation of the heterogeneous distribution of these conditions based on race.
- As race is a social construct, observed differences by race in modifiable risk factors that contribute to the development of cardiovascular disease demands further investigation into the numerous social and economic influences that underpin these findings.

INTRODUCTION

Cardiovascular disease remains the leading cause of death in the United States.[1] The disparate impact of race in influencing morbidity and mortality associated with cardiovascular disease has been well described.[2] The difference in cardiovascular disease mortality between Black and white Americans first manifests in young and middle-aged adults.[3]

Before any attempt to study the impact of race on cardiovascular disease, an appreciation for the construct of race is necessary to avoid pitfalls born of its unintended application. Race has its origins between the sixteenth and eighteenth centuries as

[a] Perelman School of Medicine, University of Pennsylvania, Philadelphia, PA, USA; [b] Penn Cardiovascular Outcomes, Quality, and Evaluative Research Center; [c] Penn Cardiovascular Center for Health Equity and Social Justice
[1] Present address: Perelman Center for Advanced Medicine, 3400 Civic Center Boulevard, 2nd Floor East, Philadelphia, PA 19104.
* Corresponding author.
E-mail address: Howard.Julien@pennmedicine.upenn.edu

Med Clin N Am 106 (2022) 401–409
https://doi.org/10.1016/j.mcna.2021.11.008
0025-7125/22/Published by Elsevier Inc.

a folk idea in English language cultures[4]; it evolved to encompass the groups of North America by the seventeenth century and gained traction in the early eighteenth century in parallel with the rise of the transatlantic slave trade. The race-based classification of people persists as a vestige from this era with no discernible genetic basis.[5] Despite the absence of a discrete genetic underpinning, societies have, and continue to, use the classification to implicitly and explicitly allocate resources and treatment creating the foundation of racism in social institutions. Consequently, the use of race in scientific literature should indicate the presence of a complex interaction of mostly social, economic, and cultural influences along with some genetic factors that have been aggregated into one variable. Some of the social, economic, and cultural influences that influence the impact of race on cardiovascular disease owe their origins to institutional, personal/perceived, and internalized racism.[6]

Epidemiology of Hyperlipidemia in Black Americans

The Centers for Disease Control and Prevention has estimated that approximately 71 million or 33.5% of US adults older than 20 years have high low-density lipoprotein cholesterol (LDL-C), whereas only 48% of those people received treatment for it and only 33% of them had their LDL-C levels less than the goal level (controlled) when treated. Education is an important indicator for pathologic LDL-C values. In populations that had not completed high school, 41% had hyperlipidemia, whereas college graduates had prevalence of only 28.7%. In addition to education, self-described race has played a large role in hyperlipidemia prevalence. The prevalence of hyperlipidemia is highest in non-Hispanic whites at 34.5%, non- Hispanic Black Americans at 30.4%, and Mexican Americans at 27.7%. These numbers are likely an underestimate because Black Americans have one of the highest uninsured rates at 11.5% and are thus less likely to receive routine cardiovascular risk factor screening.[7] In addition to lower physical activity, alcohol consumption, and diet, perceived racism may play a role in dyslipidemia within Black communities. One study conducted in 2011 showed that endorsing behavioral coping responses to perceived racism predicted higher levels of LDL-C.[8] The relationship between stress and increased LDL-C levels was not associated with other stress response systems such as cortisol, norepinephrine, epinephrine, and interleukin-6.[8] This study implies that other forms of stress may also be associated with elevated LDL-C values.

Management of Hyperlipidemia in Black Americans

Treatment of hyperlipidemia aims to reduce the risk of atherosclerotic cardiovascular disease and resultant events through reduction of LDL-C levels. The foundation of therapy is nonpharmacologic lifestyle changes. Dietary changes including reducing saturated fat, cholesterol, and alcohol intake have been shown to lower lipid blood levels. Maintaining a healthy weight as well as increasing physical activity has been shown to yield similar results.[9,10] Pharmacologic treatments of hyperlipidemia typically include statins, which inhibit cholesterol synthesis in the liver leading to lower lipid levels circulating in the blood, and are a mainstay of therapy.[11–13] Second-line lipid-lowering agents include fibrates, bile acid resins, niacin, ezetimibe, and most recently, injectable proprotein convertase subtilisin/kexin type 9 (PCSK9) inhibitors.[14] Most frequently used are ezetimibe, which is indicated with statin intolerance, and PCSK9 inhibitors, indicated when LDL-C levels remain elevated despite receiving treatment with statins along with a history of atherosclerotic cardiovascular disease.[15] When compared with non-Hispanic white Americans, black Americans have a lower prevalence of hyperlipidemia but were less likely to be treated.

Black Americans were less likely to be aware of and have their LDL-C levels controlled upon receiving treatment than their white counterparts.[16,17] Among black patients, hyperlipidemia is less likely to be controlled and has been a main contributor to cardiovascular disease and death. Despite nationwide reductions in cardiovascular disease rates black Americans continue to suffer from cardiovascular disease at greater rates than other groups. Potential solutions lie in strengthening the patient-provider relationship. Black patients are less likely to be prescribed guideline-recommended statin therapy than their white counterparts.[18] Compounding this undertreatment is a lower propensity of Black patients to trust their clinician (82.3% vs 93.8%), to believe that statin therapy is safe (36.2% vs 57.3%) or believe that it is effective (70.0% vs 74.4%), when compared with whites.

In addition, dietary changes that result in reduction of consumption of saturated fats and transfats can help lower LDL-C levels. A move toward a more plant-based diet can help manifest these changes and has been shown to be effective at lowering LDL-C levels and consequently, incidence of cardiovascular events.[19] Finally, regular forms of exercise can lower LDL-C levels. These modifiable risk factors for dyslipidemia may be particularly hard to correct considering a lack of free exercise facilities and prevalence of food deserts in urban areas.[20]

Overview of hypertension

Hypertension, defined as sustained elevated systolic blood pressure (SBP) or diastolic blood pressure (DBP), is associated with adverse clinical end points such as target organ damage, heart disease, and end-stage renal disease.[21] Although the relationship between elevated blood pressure and the risk of cardiovascular disease is continuous, SBP and DBP thresholds have been used in clinical practice to help physicians identify and treat patients at risk.[21,22] Notably, different institutions use distinct cutoffs for the clinical definition of hypertension, allowing either SBP/DBP greater than or equal to 140/90 mm Hg[23] or SBP/DBP greater than or equal to 130/80 mmHg[21,24] to signal a need for blood pressure-lowering intervention.

To measure blood pressure, modern clinical settings have generally replaced the mercury sphygmomanometer with validated electronic upper-arm cuff devices or calibrated auscultatory devices, such as aneroid sphygmomanometers.[3]

Although calibrated measurement technologies can accurately measure blood pressure in the clinic, they struggle to identify some notable manifestations of hypertension, including white coat, masked, and nocturnal hypertension.[25] White coat hypertension, a short-term and reversible increase in blood pressure, either due to the clinical environment or the presence of an observer, is not thought to be associated with cardiovascular disease.[22,26] Masked hypertension, the clinical opposite of white coat hypertension, in which patients exhibit an increased daytime ambulatory blood pressure but a normal blood pressure in clinical settings can be more dangerous and potentially prevents proper diagnosis and treatment.[22,26] Nocturnal hypertension is defined as an elevated nocturnal blood pressure (mean nocturnal SBP/DBP $\geq$120/70 mm Hg) and, like masked hypertension, is associated with increased cardiovascular disease risk.[26,27] Although these clinical presentations can each frustrate epidemiologic efforts to quantify the burden of hypertension, the rates of masked and nocturnal hypertension suggest that the true prevalence of hypertension may be underestimated. Guidance from the International Society of Hypertension (ISH) recognizes the unique challenges that these subtypes present, offering out-of-office blood pressure measurement using ambulatory blood pressure monitoring (ABPM) as a more reproducible method of diagnosing high blood pressure in patients.[25]

Epidemiology of Hypertension in Black Patients

As in other industrialized nations, hypertension is very common in the United States, with an age-adjusted prevalence estimate of 45.4% for adults older than 18 years.[24] The prevalence of hypertension is higher in men than in women (51.0% vs 39.7%) and increases with age.[24] Blacks face the highest burden of hypertension among all the racial and ethnic groups in the United States.[28] During 2017 to 2018, 57.1% of non-Hispanic Black adults had hypertension after adjusting for age compared with 43.6% of non-Hispanic whites and 50.1% of Hispanics.[24] Other estimates suggest that Black Americans consistently experience more than 10% higher prevalence of hypertension than non-Hispanic whites and Mexican Americans since 2008.[9] Disparities in hypertension between black Americans and other racial groups extend beyond prevalence estimates. Evidence suggests that black Americans develop hypertension younger and have higher recorded blood pressures than their white counterparts,[29] and National Health and Nutrition Examination Survey (NHANES) data demonstrated that differences in blood pressure can be observed between white and black women before 10 years of age.[30] The gap further widens when investigating hypertension-related deaths, with Black Americans experiencing 3 times the association between SBP and stroke risk than whites do.[9] Black Americans can expect 4.2 times the rate of end-stage renal disease and 1.5 times the rate of heart disease mortality when compared with the general population in both cases.[30] Overall, as many as 49.6% of cardiovascular disease deaths in Black males were attributable to hypertension; only 14.4% of cardiovascular disease deaths were due to hypertension among their white counterparts.[30]

In addition to traditional risk factors for hypertension, including a sedentary lifestyle, high-salt diet, and family history, researchers have proposed that racism and discrimination are associated with cardiovascular diseases and hypertension. A study showed that Blacks in areas with greater structural racism were more likely to have experienced a heart attack in the past year.[31] A random effects meta-analysis model demonstrated that perceived racial discrimination was associated with a hypertension diagnosis.[32]

Another study found that for each unit increase of racism-related vigilance, a form of anticipatory stress, Blacks faced a 4% increase in the odds of high blood pressure.[33] After accounting for other social explainers such as socioeconomic status, researchers across multiple studies found that disparities between Black and white Americans persisted, suggesting that research into other risk factors, including racism, may be needed to fully understand the observed and persistent gap in hypertension prevalence.

Although the gap in the prevalence of hypertension and associated cardiovascular diseases between Black Americans and non-Blacks in the United States is large, it is likely an underestimation. In the Jackson Heart Study, researchers showed that when using ABPM to measure daytime blood pressure, 34% of patients thought to be normotensive in a clinical evaluation were found to be hypertensive; when using daytime, nighttime, and 24-hour blood pressure from ABPM, this percentage ballooned to 52%.[26] Further research demonstrated that Black Americans with masked hypertension diagnosed via ABPM were at greater risk of a future incident clinic hypertension diagnosis than normotensive Blacks, suggesting that masked hypertension may be an intermediate step between normal and clinically high blood pressure.[34] Together, these estimates suggest that the diagnostic sensitivity of in-clinic blood pressure measurements is low and may contribute to the observed health disparities between Black Americans and their non-Black peers.

Management of Hypertension in Black Patients

Although Black patients demonstrate a greater awareness of their hypertension status and were more likely to have it treated than whites or Hispanics,[9] some estimates show that as many as 40% of self-identifying hypertensive Black Americans were not receiving antihypertensive therapy.[30] In addition, Black Americans experienced lower rates of hypertension control, which is defined as previously elevated blood pressure brought within target ranges by blood pressure-lowering interventions such as pharmaceuticals, than whites.[35,36] These estimates suggest that both un-treated and resistant hypertension play important roles in cardiovascular disease disparities experienced by Black Americans.

Common pharmacologic interventions include diuretics, calcium channel blockers (CCB), angiotensin-converting enzyme inhibitors (ACEI), angiotensin II receptor blockers (ARB), and β-blockers. Although each of these drugs can lower blood pressure in the general population, studies have shown that some drugs confer more modest reductions in blood pressure in Black Americans than in whites.[36] A meta-analysis of studies with ACEI monotherapy showed that the average Black patient had a final SBP/DBP blood pressure that was 4.6/2.8 mm Hg higher than that of white patients.[36] In addition, ACEI/ARB treatment has been demonstrated to be less effective in Black patients than other drug treatment classes.[23,36,37] Angioedema, an adverse drug effect of ACEI therapy, seems to occur as much as 3 times more often in black patients than non-Black patients,[38] but with a general population risk of ACEI-associated angioedema of less than 1%, it is unclear to what degree this difference should impact clinical decision making.[25,36] Interpreting these data with the knowledge that race is a social construct calls for additional research to determine the biological factors responsible for these differences. These findings have inspired differential recommendations for first-line therapy in Black versus non-Black populations; the Joint National Committee (JNC) 8 recommends ACEI or ARBs as options for initial antihypertension treatment in non-Blacks but drops these suggestions when considering Black patients.[23]

Differences in drug responses have sparked investigations into causal pathways of hypertension in Black Americans, such as increased dietary sodium sensitivity and low renin levels.[36] These theories imply that genetic differences can simultaneously explain increased rates of hypertension as well as reduced responses to therapy, but a genetic explanation of these observed and perceived differences has yet to be clearly identified. Studies that quantified ancestry using models that characterize genomic similarity suggest no association between West African ancestry and nocturnal hypertension or reduced hypertension control.[27,39] Importantly, studies have shown that known genetic factors for hypertension together explain less than 3% of observed individual differences[39]; other environmental factors, such as access to affordable health care and healthy food, likely play a larger role in the significant and persistent disparities faced by Black Americans over the past 20 years and beyond.

The emphasis on the effects of individual drugs also distracts from the well-established benefits of multidrug therapy in hypertension control. Monotherapy with ACEI and ARB treatment did not significantly increase odds of hypertension control in Black Americans,[37] but when combined with other treatments such as diuretics or CCB, they provided even stronger clinical benefits in blood pressure reduction than any drug individually.[23,25,30,35–37] It is estimated that if dosages for antihypertensives were increased on 1 of 3 visits with observed elevated blood pressure, hypertension control would increase from 45% to 66% in a single year.[40] Indeed, the Kaiser Permanente Southern California health system, implementing strategies like treatment intensification to increase dosages and combine drugs, raised the rate of hypertension control among Black patients to more than 80%, simultaneously cutting the previous gap with whites by 50% and suggesting that hypertension control can be better achieved with team-based approaches to disease management and flexible treatment strategies rather than forms of genetic scapegoating.[26,41]

Behavioral interventions are a critical tool in combating hypertension. The Dietary Approaches to Stop Hypertension (DASH) diet, similar to the Mediterranean diet, has been shown to lower SBP by as much as 11 mm Hg, a reduction that mirrors the effects of some antihypertensive drugs.[29,35,42] In spite of these purported benefits, adherence to the DASH-type diet among hypertensive adults in the United States has steadily decreased over the past few decades, especially in Black American populations.[29,42] Challenges to adherence include DASH's limited integration with the cultural practices of Black communities as well as poor guidance on specific steps required for implementation, such as recipe modifications and grocery shopping.[42] Although diet and other individual changes, such as regular exercise, are known to reduce blood pressure in hypertensive patients, these challenges and others faced by Black Americans are influenced by community-level conditions, such as access to health care. Community outreach efforts such as barbershop engagement has had notable success in studies, with one project achieving a mean SBP reduction of 27.0 mm Hg from a baseline mean SBP of 152.8 mm Hg.[43]

SUMMARY

A modern approach to mitigating the impact of cardiovascular disease on Americans demands not only an understanding of modifiable conditions that contribute to its development but also a greater appreciation of the heterogeneous distribution of these conditions based on race. As race is not a biological construct, further research is needed to fully elucidate the mechanisms that contribute to these differences.

The consequences of the differential impact of modifiable risk factors on cardiovascular disease outcomes among Black Americans compared with white Americans cannot be understated. Because race is a social construct, observed differences by race in modifiable risk factors that contribute to the development of cardiovascular disease demands further investigation into the numerous social and economic influences that underpin these findings.

CLINICS CARE POINTS

- The prevalence of hyperlipidemia is highest in non-Hispanic whites at 34.5%, non-Hispanic Black Americans at 30.4%, and Mexican Americans at 27.7% though these data likely underestimate prevalence in Black Americans who have one of the highest uninsured rates in America.

- Black patients are less likely to be prescribed guideline-recommended statin therapy than their white counterparts.

- Blacks face the highest burden of hypertension among all the racial and ethnic groups in the United States.

- Black Americans develop hypertension younger and have higher recorded blood pressures than their white counterparts.

DISCLOSURE

The authors have nothing to disclose.

REFERENCES

1. Prevention. CfDCa. Underlying Cause of Death, 1999–2018. CDC WONDER On-line Database. 2018.
2. Writing Group M, Mozaffarian D, Benjamin EJ, et al. American Heart Association Statistics C and Stroke Statistics S. Heart Disease and Stroke Statistics-2016 Up-date: A Report From the American Heart Association. Circulation 2016;133: e38–360.
3. Jolly S, Vittinghoff E, Chattopadhyay A, et al. Higher cardiovascular disease prev-alence and mortality among younger blacks compared to whites. Am J Med 2010;123:811–8.
4. Smedley A, Smedley BD. Race as biology is fiction, racism as a social problem is real: Anthropological and historical perspectives on the social construction of race. Am Psychol 2005;60:16–26.
5. Ioannidis JPA, Powe NR, Yancy C. Recalibrating the Use of Race in Medical Research. JAMA 2021;325:623–4.
6. Wyatt SB, Williams DR, Calvin R, et al. Racism and cardiovascular disease in Af-rican Americans. Am J Med Sci 2003;325:315–31.
7. Artiga S. Changes in Health Coverage by Race and Ethnicity since the ACA, 2010-2018. 2020;2021. Available at: https://files.kff.org/attachment/Issue-Brief-Changes-in-Health-Coverage-by-Race-and-Ethnicity-since-the-ACA-2010-2018.pdf.
8. Mwendwa DT, Sims RC, Madhere S, et al. The influence of coping with perceived racism and stress on lipid levels in African Americans. J Natl Med Assoc 2011; 103:594–601.
9. Carnethon MR, Pu J, Howard G, et al, American Heart Association Council on E, Prevention, Council on Cardiovascular Disease in the Y, Council on C, Stroke N, Council on Clinical C, Council on Functional G, Translational B and Stroke C. Car-diovascular Health in African Americans: A Scientific Statement From the Amer-ican Heart Association. Circulation 2017;136:e393–423.
10. Koutsari C, Karpe F, Humphreys SM, et al. Exercise prevents the accumulation of triglyceride-rich lipoproteins and their remnants seen when changing to a high-carbohydrate diet. Arterioscler Thromb Vasc Biol 2001;21:1520–5.
11. Stone NJ, Robinson JG, Lichtenstein AH, et al. Tomaselli GF and American Col-lege of Cardiology/American Heart Association Task Force on Practice G. 2013 ACC/AHA guideline on the treatment of blood cholesterol to reduce atheroscle-rotic cardiovascular risk in adults: a report of the American College of Cardiol-ogy/American Heart Association Task Force on Practice Guidelines. Circulation 2014;129:S1–45.
12. Cholesterol Treatment Trialists C, Mihaylova B, Emberson J, et al. The effects of lowering LDL cholesterol with statin therapy in people at low risk of vascular dis-ease: meta-analysis of individual data from 27 randomised trials. Lancet 2012; 380:581–90.
13. Taylor F, Ward K, Moore TH, et al. Statins for the primary prevention of cardiovas-cular disease. Cochrane Database Syst Rev 2011;(1):CD004816.
14. Grundy SM, Stone NJ, Bailey AL, et al. 2018 AHA/ACC/AACVPR/AAPA/ABC/ACPM/ADA/AGS/APhA/ASPC/NLA/PCNA Guideline on the Management of Blood Cholesterol: A Report of the American College of Cardiology/American Heart

Association Task Force on Clinical Practice Guidelines. Circulation 2019;139: e1082–143.

15. Giugliano RP, Sabatine MS. Are PCSK9 Inhibitors the Next Breakthrough in the Cardiovascular Field? J Am Coll Cardiol 2015;65:2638–51.

16. Massing MW, Foley KA, Carter-Edwards L, et al. Disparities in lipid management for African Americans and Caucasians with coronary artery disease: a national cross-sectional study. BMC Cardiovasc Disord 2004;4:15.

17. Zweifler RM, McClure LA, Howard VJ, et al. Racial and geographic differences in prevalence, awareness, treatment and control of dyslipidemia: the reasons for geographic and racial differences in stroke (REGARDS) study. Neuroepidemiology 2011;37:39–44.

18. Nanna MG, Navar AM, Zakroysky P, et al. Association of patient perceptions of cardiovascular risk and beliefs on statin drugs with racial differences in statin use: insights from the patient and provider assessment of lipid management registry. JAMA Cardiol 2018;3:739–48.

19. Clifton PM. Diet, exercise and weight loss and dyslipidaemia. Pathology 2019;51: 222–6.

20. Kelli HM, Hammadah M, Ahmed H, et al. Association between living in food deserts and cardiovascular risk. Circ Cardiovasc Qual Outcomes 2017;10:e003532.

21. Whelton PK, Carey RM, Aronow WS, et al. 2017 ACC/AHA/AAPA/ABC/ACPM/ AGS/APhA/ASH/ASPC/NMA/PCNA Guideline for the Prevention, Detection, Evaluation, and Management of High Blood Pressure in Adults: A Report of the American College of Cardiology/American Heart Association Task Force on Clinical Practice Guidelines. Hypertension 2018;71:e13–115.

22. Staessen JA, Wang J, Bianchi G, et al. Essential hypertension. Lancet 2003;361: 1629–41.

23. James PA, Oparil S, Carter BL, et al. 2014 evidence-based guideline for the management of high blood pressure in adults: report from the panel members appointed to the Eighth Joint National Committee (JNC 8). JAMA 2014;311:507–20.

24. Ostchega Y, Fryar CD, Nwankwo T, et al. Hypertension Prevalence Among Adults Aged 18 and Over: United States, 2017-2018. NCHS Data Brief 2020;(364):1–8.

25. Unger T, Borghi C, Charchar F, et al. 2020 International Society of Hypertension Global Hypertension Practice Guidelines. Hypertension 2020;75:1334–57.

26. Muntner P, Abdalla M, Correa A, et al. Hypertension in blacks: unanswered questions and future directions for the JHS (Jackson Heart Study). Hypertension 2017; 69:761–9.

27. Booth JN III, Li M, Shimbo D, et al. West African Ancestry and Nocturnal Blood Pressure in African Americans: The Jackson Heart Study. Am J Hypertens 2018;31:706–14.

28. Kramer H, Han C, Post W, et al. Racial/ethnic differences in hypertension and hypertension treatment and control in the multi-ethnic study of atherosclerosis (MESA). Am J Hypertens 2004;17:963–70.

29. Go AS, Mozaffarian D, Roger VL, et al. American Heart Association Statistics C and Stroke Statistics S. Heart disease and stroke statistics–2013 update: a report from the American Heart Association. Circulation 2013;127:e6–245.

30. Ferdinand KC, Saunders E. Hypertension-related morbidity and mortality in African Americans–why we need to do better. J Clin Hypertens (Greenwich) 2006;8: 21–30.

31. Lukachko A, Hatzenbuehler ML, Keyes KM. Structural racism and myocardial infarction in the United States. Soc Sci Med 2014;103:42–50.

32. Dolezsar CM, McGrath JJ, Herzig AJM, et al. Perceived racial discrimination and hypertension: a comprehensive systematic review. Health Psychol 2014;33: 20–34.

33. Hicken MT, Lee H, Morenoff J, et al. Racial/ethnic disparities in hypertension prevalence: reconsidering the role of chronic stress. Am J Public Health 2014; 104:117–23.

34. Abdalla M, Booth JN 3rd, Seals SR, et al. Masked hypertension and incident clinic hypertension among blacks in the Jackson Heart Study. Hypertension 2016;68:220–6.

35. Ferdinand K, Batieste T, Fleurestil M. Contemporary and future concepts on hypertension in African Americans: COVID-19 and Beyond. J Natl Med Assoc 2020;112:315–23.

36. Helmer A, Slater N, Smithgall S. A Review of ACE Inhibitors and ARBs in black patients with hypertension. Ann Pharmacother 2018;52:1143–51.

37. Clemmer JS, Pruett WA, Lirette ST. Racial and sex differences in the response to first-line antihypertensive therapy. Front Cardiovasc Med 2020;7:608037.

38. Kostis JB, Kim HJ, Rusnak J, et al. Incidence and characteristics of angioedema associated with enalapril. Arch Intern Med 2005;165:1637–42.

39. Rao S, Segar MW, Bress AP, et al. Association of Genetic West African Ancestry, Blood Pressure Response to Therapy, and Cardiovascular Risk Among Self-Reported Black Individuals in the Systolic Blood Pressure Reduction Intervention Trial (SPRINT). JAMA Cardiol 2020;6(4):388–98.

40. Okonofua EC, Simpson KN, Jesri A, et al. Therapeutic inertia is an impediment to achieving the Healthy People 2010 blood pressure control goals. Hypertension 2006;47:345–51.

41. Bartolome RE, Chen A, Handler J, et al. Population care management and team-based approach to reduce racial disparities among African Americans/Blacks with Hypertension. Perm J 2016;20:53–9.

42. Scisney-Matlock M, Bosworth HB, Giger JN, et al. Strategies for implementing and sustaining therapeutic lifestyle changes as part of hypertension management in African Americans. Postgrad Med 2009;121:147–59.

43. Victor RG, Lynch K, Li N, et al. A cluster-randomized trial of blood-pressure reduction in black barbershops. N Engl J Med 2018;378:1291–301.

Moving?

Make sure your subscription moves with you!

To notify us of your new address, find your **Clinics Account Number** (located on your mailing label above your name), and contact customer service at:

Email: journalscustomerservice-usa@elsevier.com

800-654-2452 (subscribers in the U.S. & Canada)
314-447-8871 (subscribers outside of the U.S. & Canada)

Fax number: 314-447-8029

Elsevier Health Sciences Division
Subscription Customer Service
3251 Riverport Lane
Maryland Heights, MO 63043

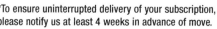

*To ensure uninterrupted delivery of your subscription, please notify us at least 4 weeks in advance of move.

ELSEVIER